AFTA SpringerBriefs in Family Therapy

Series Editor
Carmen Knudson-Martin
Education & Counseling, Rogers Hall
Lewis & Clark Grad School
Portland, OR, USA

SpringerBriefs present concise summaries of cutting-edge research and practical applications. Featuring compact volumes of 50 to 125 pages, the series covers a range of content from professional to academic. Typical topics might include: A timely report of state-of-the art analytical techniques A bridge between new research results, as published in journal articles, and a contextual literature review A snapshot of a hot or emerging topic An in-depth case study or clinical example A presentation of core concepts that students must understand in order to make independent contributions

Lindsey A. Nice • Christie Eppler

Editors

Social Justice and Systemic Family Therapy Training

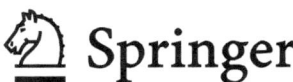 Springer

Editors
Lindsey A. Nice
Pacific Lutheran University
Tacoma, WA, USA

Christie Eppler 🆔
Couples and Family Therapy
Seattle University
Seattle, WA, USA

ISSN 2196-5528   ISSN 2196-5536   (electronic)
AFTA SpringerBriefs in Family Therapy
ISBN 978-3-031-29929-2   ISBN 978-3-031-29930-8   (eBook)
https://doi.org/10.1007/978-3-031-29930-8

This Springer imprint is published by the registered company Springer Nature Switzerland AG
The registered company address is: Gewerbestrasse 11, 6330 Cham, Switzerland

Series Foreword

The AFTA Springer Briefs in Family Therapy is an official publication of the American Family Therapy Academy. Each volume focuses on the practice and policy implications of innovative systemic research and theory in family therapy and allied fields. Our goal is to make information about families and systemic practices in societal contexts widely accessible in a reader friendly, conversational, and practical style. AFTA's core commitment to equality, social responsibility, and justice are represented in each volume.

With growing awareness of the damaging effects of social inequities on personal and relational well-being, systemic therapy training programs are increasingly called upon to teach in ways that promote social justice. Mission statements change to target these values. Accreditation standards require programs to document that they do so. More and more, scholarship in the field examines clinical issues and practices through a social justice lens and curriculums change. But there is very little guidance for how to apply social justice principles in family therapy teaching or what this means day to day in the classroom. *Social Justice and Systemic Family Therapy Training* does just this. Editors Lindsey Nice and Christie Eppler invited a richly diverse group of educators to share their experiences as they move from theory about social justice to living it.

The authors of each chapter generously share pivotal moments of difficult conversations, personal and professional vulnerabilities, and challenging choices as they shift toward intentionally embodying social justice in how they teach and relate to students and colleagues. Readers will be left with a realistic, inspirational, and deeply personal sense of the challenges and opportunities that arise when stepping toward increased awareness of social justice in every aspect of training. Like me, you will be grateful for their courage in sharing their missteps and struggles along the way and benefit from the wisdom gleaned from their stories and suggestions.

Carmen Knudson-Martin, Series Editor
AFTA Springer Briefs in Family Therapy
Portland, Oregon

AFTA Springer Briefs in Family Therapy

A publication of the American Family Therapy Academy
Founded in 1977, the **American Family Therapy Academy** is a non-profit organization of leading family therapy teachers, clinicians, program directors, policymakers, researchers, and social scientists dedicated to advancing systemic thinking and practices for families in their social context.

Vision

AFTA envisions a just world by transforming social contexts that promote health, safety, and well-being of all families and communities.

Mission

AFTA's mission is developing, researching, teaching, and disseminating progressive, just family therapy and family-centered practices and policies.

Acknowledgements and Thanks

We are grateful to the many people who've supported the creation of this book. We especially thank our colleagues who've sat with us through hours of conversation, and who both challenge and support us. In particular, we want to thank Dr. David Ward, Dr. Elisabeth Esmiol Wilson, Dr. Jessica ChenFeng, and Dr. Lana Kim (Lindsey), and Dr. Jeanette Rodriguez, Dr. Erica Martin, Dr. Rebecca (Becky) Cobb, Dr. Ashley Hicks, Dr. Martha Morgan, and LaDonna Smith (Christie).

We also want to thank our students. From my (Lindsey's) early conception of a chapter where student voices were included, to the courage and vulnerability we see time and time again as students engage with each other around these topics and connect across differences, we are reminded of how we are changed as much (or more) as we impact students.

We appreciate the support from our respective institutions: Pacific Lutheran University (Lindsey) and Seattle University (Christie). This book began as a project during my (Lindsey's) sabbatical year, and I'm thankful to have been provided an opportunity to take time for my own professional development in this way.

We want to thank Melissa Carter, a graduate assistant and student at Pacific Lutheran University, who helped us with final edits and formatting in preparation for this volume's submission for publication. Her support over these past few months has been invaluable.

This book would not have materialized without the important contributions of each chapter's authors. We are so grateful for the variety of experiences captured in each chapter. Writing for this book came at a particularly difficult time, during the aftermath of Covid-19, throughout continued violence against people of Color, and the Supreme Court's overturning of Roe v. Wade. We've deeply appreciated the heart and time commitments each author contributed during so many larger social difficulties.

We've long appreciated the professional home that the American Family Therapy Academy provides, and are thankful to Dr. Carmen Knudson-Martin for her guidance both professionally as an early career academic (Lindsey) and with this book.

Lastly, we want to thank our families and loved ones. I, (Lindsey), want to especially thank my husband Aaron, for his commitment to creating an equitable and mutually supportive home with me, and for all his encouragement and care throughout the creation of this book. And to our three children, Lucy, Andy, and Rory: I hope you always remember that love looks like justice. I, (Christie), thank my family, circle of friends, wise storytellers, and Luke and Mossy. I dedicate this text to those who struggle and strive to create a more just and humane world.

Contents

Contributors

Branson Boykins Alliant International University, San Diego, CA, USA

Jessica ChenFeng Fuller Theological Seminary, Pasadena, CA, USA

Wonyoung Cho Lewis & Clark College, Portland, OR, USA

Justine D'Arrigo California State University, San Bernardino, CA, USA

Lana Kim Lewis & Clark College, Portland, OR, USA

Nicki King Pacific Lutheran University, Tacoma, WA, USA

Matthew R. Mock JFK School of Psychology of National University, Pleasant Hill, CA, USA

Martha L. Morgan Gobert UMass Global, Irvine, CA, USA

Lindsey A. Nice Pacific Lutheran University, Tacoma, WA, USA

Anthony Pennant Antioch University, Seattle, CA, USA

Gabriela Raisl Pacific Lutheran University, Tacoma, WA, USA

Sarah K. Samman Alliant International University, San Diego, CA, USA

Jennifer M. Sampson Antioch University, Seattle, WA, USA

Zain Shamoon Antioch University, Seattle, CA, USA

Elisabeth Esmiol Wilson Pacific Lutheran University, Tacoma, WA, USA
NW Reflections Counseling, Puyallup, WA, USA

About the Editors

Lindsey A. Nice, PhD, LMFT is program chair of the Marriage and Family Therapy Department and an associate professor at Pacific Lutheran University in Tacoma, WA. Before becoming an MFT, she worked as a nurse at a small hospital in Oregon and still enjoys learning about the intersection of physical, mental, and relational health. Her research interests include the development of contextually-sensitive and socially-just pedagogy, religion and spirituality in therapy, medical family therapy, and partner relational equity. In addition to teaching, she has a small private practice and especially enjoys working with couples and parents of young children. Lindsey is a previous co-editor on another AFTA Springer Brief: *Socially Just Religious and Spiritual Interventions: Ethical Uses of Therapeutic Power.* When away from work, she enjoys spending time with her husband Aaron and their three pre-school aged children: Lucy, Andy, and Rory, on their 1930's six-acre farm in the foothills of Mt. Rainier.

Christie Eppler, PhD, LMFT is a program director and professor in Couples and Family Therapy at Seattle University. Her research areas include systemic resilience, narrative family therapy, and promoting social justice in relationship therapy. Christie's studies have been published in the *Journal of Marital and Family Therapy*, *Journal of Systemic Therapy*, *Feminist Family Therapy*, and *Journal of Family Psychotherapy*. She presents regularly at American Association of Marriage and Family Therapy's (AAMFT) National Conferences. Christie is an AAMFT Approved Supervisor and a Licensed Marriage and Family Therapist (LMFT; Washington). Christie teaches ethics, assessment, and group supervision classes. She enjoys helping new interns mitigate their anxieties while utilizing systems models and common factors to conceptualize clients. Clinically, Christie works from a critically conscious, strength-based, narrative family therapy approach. Her own resilient-care practices include running marathons, practicing yoga, and hiking with Mossy where the forest meets the sea.

Welcoming "Not Yet": Personal, Professional, and Political Changes in the Classroom

Lindsey A. Nice, Nicki King, and Gabriela Raisl

1 Introduction

Each evening around 7:00, I (Lindsey) have two wiggly toddlers, wet hair from their bath, clean pajamas on, cuddle up next to me as we read books together before bed. One of their favorites is called *The Day You Begin* (Woodson, 2018). In it, a classroom full of kids from all kinds of different life experiences get to know one another. There are some lines toward the end that read:

There will be times when the world feels like a place that you're standing all the way outside of... and all that stands beside you is your own brave self – steady as steel and ready even though you don't yet know what you're ready for. There will be times when you walk into a room and no one there is quite like you until the day you begin to share your stories. And all at once, in the room where no one else is quite like you, the world opens itself up a little wider to make some space for you. (p. 32).

I think often about that last line, and what it means to make space for people to belong – in particular, my students – in the classroom, and how powerful those relational connections can be in a world that feels so polarized. In his book, *The Enduring, Invisible, Ubiquitous Centrality of Whiteness* (2022), Ken Hardy describes how a focus on "product" over "process" (p. 20) reflects the centrality of whiteness in so many spaces. In academia, most systemic therapy programs have focused some effort on recruiting students of Color and increasing "cultural awareness": limited, stereotypic descriptions of how to work with different groups of people (often from a white-therapist perspective). These are examples of "product" ways of thinking that only impact change on a very superficial level.

L. A. Nice (✉) · N. King · G. Raisl
Pacific Lutheran University, Tacoma, WA, USA
e-mail: nicela@plu.edu

© American Family Therapy Academy (AFTA) 2023
L. A. Nice, C. Eppler (eds.), *Social Justice and Systemic Family Therapy Training*,
AFTA SpringerBriefs in Family Therapy, https://doi.org/10.1007/978-3-031-29930-8_1

"Process" changes are more difficult: they require a shift in epistemology (Hardy, 2022). This involves changing the academic system itself: closely evaluating the white ideologies, principles, and values that often serve as a foundation for the theories we teach (who was afforded the opportunity to research, publish, and become known as the "expert?"), the materials we require students to read (whose voices are privileged or marginalized, and in what other non-academic spaces – community groups, blogs, podcasts, etc. – is valuable information available?), the ways we ask them to sit with clients (who defines "professionalism?"), how we evaluate them (prioritizing individual growth over group processes), and who they see represented in positions of power (predominantly white people).

Early social justice educators helped initiate this shift away from "product" toward "process" by explicitly incorporating conversations about intersectional identities with trainees to help them understand both their own areas of privilege or marginalization, and the oppressive factors impacting clients' lives (McGoldrick et al., 1999). Others emphasized the need for contextual exploration across all courses and highlighted ways to move people who have been on the margins toward the center (McDowell & Shelton, 2002). More recently, educators continue to engage in "tough and transformative conversations" (Eppler, 2021) about the centrality of whiteness in leadership (Hardy, 2022; Quek & Hsieh, 2021), the struggles of faculty of Color (Hardy & McGoldrick, 2019; Quek & Hsieh, 2021), and the painful, often re-traumatizing experiences of students of Color (Allan & Singh Poulsen, 2017; Hardy & Bobes, 2016).

While there is a growing body of literature on the importance of addressing diversity, equity, and inclusion more adequately in systemic training programs, most of what exists emphasizes classroom processes with a focus on what students need to learn to be more contextually aware. Relatively little research addresses the experiences of family therapy educators as we try to put these principles into practice in teaching. When my co-editor Christie and I began working on this volume, one of the things we continued to circle back to was the hope that this would be a collection of these experiences, rather than a "how-to" guide, shared by systemic therapy educators. To this end, we asked chapter authors to share two or three moments of impact in teaching that supported increased awareness of social justice issues: times when there was a connection and growth, or times when there was a "miss" and a need for repair. In this volume, authors described shifts at three different levels:

1. Personal: interactions with students that create better understanding of issues of power.
2. Professional: interactions with colleagues that provide support and accountability.
3. Political: interventions aimed at changing the larger academic institution.

Through each of their stories runs the common thread of the importance of relationships: justice is inherently relational! It is in these "in between" spaces that we continue to be changed. We are so grateful to the authors whose voices are included in this text: systemic educators and clinicians who have committed themselves to cultivating diverse learning communities where equity and inclusion are prioritized.

Please note that throughout this book, each chapter reflects the capitalization of "people of Color," "Black," "white," etc., preferred by that chapter author. We hope that in reading their stories, you too will feel supported and encouraged, as we have, in working toward a more just academic and therapeutic landscape.

In this chapter, my co-authors (two of my students, Nicki and Gaby) and I will reflect on a classroom experience that changed all three of us in different ways and moved me as an educator toward more equitable, anti-racist teaching practices. This created a ripple across each of the above levels of change: we were each changed personally, it impacted my conversations with colleagues (professional change), and lastly it changed the way I teach that class (political change). You will hear about this experience from each of our perspectives, and we will summarize some of the themes that surfaced during this process: the helpfulness of a "not yet" approach to learning, the relationship between white supremacy and perfectionism, and the importance of nuanced, relationship-grounded repairing conversations.

2 My Identities: Lindsey

I am now in my tenth year of teaching at a small, liberal-arts university in Washington state. The university sits in an interesting location, wedged between the more urban, liberal city of Tacoma, and the very rural, conservative towns that skirt Mt. Rainier. Our MFT program is compact, with only three faculty members, a number of contract supervisors, and a cohort of about 20 students who join us each year. Until May 2022, we had been a group of three white faculty; we have since hired two new faculty, one Black man and one Chinese-American woman, who joined us in Fall 2022. The murder of George Floyd in 2020 deeply impacted us as a program, and I look back now on that as the beginning of a shift away from a "diversity" model toward an explicitly anti-racist, anti-sexist, anti-homophobic culture.

In addition to being a teacher, I am also a wife, a mom, and the descendent of Scottish, Irish, and German immigrants. My husband and I live on a small farm with our 3.5-year-old, 2-year-old, and a new baby who came into our family just 1 month ago. My faith is another significant part of my identity. I grew up a fourth-generation Seventh-day Adventist and have gone through many iterations of my faith, especially in the last 5 years. When it no longer felt congruent to attend a church where women could not be ordained, we began remotely joining an SDA off-shoot church in California that is explicitly social-justice oriented. It has felt healing to us in many ways to connect with a group where spiritual leadership is mostly people of Color, queer folks, and women.

3 Background of Experiences

One of my recent teaching experiences (Fall 2022) directly shaped some new under-standings of myself, others, and socially just teaching in the classroom. In 2020, our university published a series of seven actions toward institutional equity and anti-racist practices, meant to help move us from goals toward actionable change. These included specific interventions like changing our hiring processes, creating a culture of "critical care" that interrupts our culture of "busy," undoing policies that have had a disproportionately harmful impact on faculty and students of Color, and revising curricula to decenter whiteness. During our faculty retreat that fall, we reviewed these principles and talked in-depth about ways we could integrate them into our MFT program.

One of the courses I taught for the first time was our introduction to systems theory concepts for the incoming cohort. I significantly revised the syllabus to include a substantial amount of reading from experts of Color, including a week on "emotional regulation in social justice work." I had two readings for that day, both written primarily by women of Color. We talked about context and identities in ses-sion from a power-aware perspective, ways that emotions can prompt us to contrib-ute unwittingly to oppression, can intervene in our ability to see and resist oppression, and can also fuel resistance to oppression (Garcia et al., 2015), and ways in which we can empathize with others, even those who represent groups of people who have been harmful to us historically.

In an activity based on one of the readings, I asked students in small groups to think about some scenario questions on power, and how their own intersecting iden-tities impact emotional regulation when it comes to caring about power and how this impacts clients' lives. The reflection prompt at the end was "what will help me most in learning to regulate my emotions (by naming and validating, and responding authentically) when I notice big feelings coming up in therapy?" As groups were forming and discussions began happening around the room, two students (my co-authors, Gaby and Nicki) – both women of Color – raised their hands and asked me to come over to their group. They expressed feeling some hesitance about this activ-ity and believed this stemmed from it centering a white experience of what it means to be empathetic in session.

I was not sure what to do next. I knew this would probably be (or need to be) an in-depth discussion, and small groups were already in-progress. I did not know if I should pause them and bring us all together, or wait and have a conversation with Gaby and Nicki on our own (I worried this would feel like a dismissal). I also found myself thinking ahead and worrying about where this could go; I knew as a white faculty member, I probably had some blind spots around this and wanted to know what Gaby and Nicki were feeling. I also felt strongly that the initial message I had been trying to get across through the readings and activity was important; that we should (and this has to be nuanced, of course) be able to empathize with people who are different from us.

I ended up not stopping the small groups already in-progress, but asked Gaby and Nicki if we could talk more about what they were saying at the end of the activity when everyone could be involved. For context, about half of the group were people of Color, about half were white, and about 1/3 identified as queer or non-binary/gender non-conforming. As I listened and asked questions, the disconnect between my intent and impact became clear. While my intent had been to acknowledge how our lived experiences impact our emotional bandwidth for empathizing with clients who are harmful or represent harmful systems, the message students of Color heard was "no matter the situation, your job is to show up with empathy and validate." This felt like a "coddling" of the hurt being perpetuated, and like I was asking them to be scapegoats for accountability, when people of Color are already asked to take care of whites in so many other contexts (Hardy, 2022).

This conversation, and another that followed between Gaby, Nicki, and myself, was one of the most impactful of my teaching career. Gaby shared, "I can't do empathy without vulnerability, and asking me to empathize (and therefore be further vulnerable) may not be safe. Empathizing feels like perpetuating this image of a Black woman I can't be… a Mamie figure who just smiles and takes it. There are so many layers to this servitude of self that I already experience. Sometimes I feel like the 'giving tree' that is expected to be happy to just be left as a stump." Nicki reflected, "As women of Color, we already know how to regulate our emotions… we have to do that all the time just to get through the day." Gaby added, "I won't agree with the opinions of all people of Color. So just because those articles were written by women of Color doesn't mean I'll agree with them or that they represent my experience."

Of course, I thought, all of that makes sense! The problem was not that empathy was not an important issue for therapists from marginalized backgrounds; it was that the process and issues involved might be different, and that the way I had presented the assignment framed all students as coming from a place of some power. As I allowed myself to let go of my fear around being wrong, being found out, being called out, etc., I stepped into a both/and space where I could hold onto myself (stopping myself from going into perfectionistic shame and fragility) and also hear the impact I had had on students. It felt very important in that moment that I be able to do both of these simultaneously for us to move toward better understanding and connection. I continue to be grateful to Gaby and Nicki for their courage and emotional fortitude in coming forward with me, a white professor, when I am sure this was one of many situations they had encountered with someone in authority who "didn't get it."

4   Lessons Learned

4.1   "Not Yet"

One of the phrases I keep mentally coming back to as I try to stay engaged in dismantling my own biases and "isms" is "not yet." My tendency in the past has been to stay in a very "either/or" place when confronted with something that challenges me. I felt (and often still feel) the need to immediately make a decision about whether something is right or wrong, valid or invalid: "I don't understand that, so it must be wrong;" "That's not my lived experience, so it must not be true." I am working on allowing myself time to process things, especially with other folks who are similarly invested in this work, before arriving at any sort of conclusion. I have a sticky note taped to my computer with the phrase "not yet" to help remind myself of this when I feel pulled to that place. Instead of "I don't understand that, so it must be wrong," I'm working on reminding myself: "I don't understand that – yet." That "yet" feels like a powerful reminder that (1) I am allowed to be wrong, (2) I am allowed to not know something, and (3) I am allowed to change over time.

That requires me to continue to do a lot of my own work around unpacking how those original assumptions came to be. In so many relationships in my own life, there was always a winner and a loser in each argument: a view supported by the dominant culture which emphasizes individual, competition, and power-over (Hardy, 2022). I rarely saw anyone say "I'm sorry," and there seemed to be great shame in being wrong about something. These patterns make seeing things from someone else's perspective difficult, which, of course, mirrored the process happening in class that day. I needed to be able to see things from my students' perspectives, which were widely varied across the room, instead of my own. I was asking them to hold empathy, when what really needed to happen was for me to hold empathy for them.

4.2   Perfectionism as a Symptom of White Supremacy

Perfectionism has impacted me in some deeply harmful ways. I still remember a conversation with the chair of our department during my first year of teaching: I sat down in his office in tears, having just received my second set of teaching evaluations, and was wondering if I was cut out for this work. His gentle response back to me was, "have you struggled with perfectionism?" I had not had anyone name it quite like that before, and I realized how deeply rooted the need to be "right," and "good," and "enough" was within me. As I have worked on this in my own therapy, part of my unpacking has been around the connections between perfectionism and my white identity. I have long since let go of the idea that perfectionism is any sort of "trait" that I was born with. Perfectionism is deeply embedded in white supremacist culture that tells us we cannot be whole; we cannot show up in all of our human messiness, and we cannot acknowledge our mistakes.

This kind of perfectionism directly supports racism. In her book, *Why Are All the Black Kids Sitting Together in the Cafeteria? Conversations About Race,* Beverly Daniel Tatum (2017) says, "if we wait for perfection… we will never break the silence. The cycle of racism will continue uninterrupted." Perfectionism shows up in the classroom in all sorts of insidious ways that look like respectability politics and tone policing (Kendall, 2020). For me, it looked like my fear of being called out in front of students, and not having the "right" answer. My harmful impact on students was that this put them (in particular, my two co-authors) in a place of having to clean up my perfectionistic mess! This is something that never should have been on them in the first place. In one of her podcasts (2020), Catherine Pugh reflects, "What you do is not called 'help' when it is your mess we are cleaning." Perfectionism and its link to white supremacy is for me to continue to work on.

5   Nicki

I am a second-year graduate student in a Marriage and Family Therapy program. I just recently retired from childcare, which has been my profession for the past 10 years. Aside from being a grad student, I am also a wife and mother of two. I am a 40-year-old cisgender woman, who is half black/half white, and I identify as mixed race, bi-racial, and African American. My husband is white. Together we are trying to help navigate our mixed-race children through the racial constructs of our society, while keeping lines of communication open around race, anti-hate, anti-racism, and white supremacy. As I write this, our children are just about to turn nine and eleven. Other important aspects of my identity include being the oldest of five sisters, growing up in a feminist household, and different periods of belonging to both Methodist and Seventh-day Adventist faiths.

Growing up in an affluent area of North Tacoma and attending school in Fircrest (a small, mostly White suburb of Tacoma) meant being immersed in White culture, White-centered experiences, and learning about White-centered curriculum taught by all White educators in a predominately White institution. I was one of very few interracial or African American students and one of even fewer African American girls in most of my social settings and educational spaces growing up. Learning how to regulate my emotions as a young child was imperative so that I did not receive unwanted or harsher treatment than my White counterparts. Being aware of my intersectionalities and how my visible identities were different from the majority of my peers helped to keep me safer in these predominantly White spaces. My own experiences mirror so many others: seeing children of color treated as older than they are, and therefore having more responsibility thrust upon them than their White counterparts. In different situations, when emotions run high, keeping their feelings and emotions "in check," so to speak, is vital to the outcome of the situation and the treatment or consequence directed at that child, often to an extent beyond what they should be managing at their age. Most people of color can relate to this importance and the need for emotional regulation for safety purposes.

In Fall 2021, during a group exercise in Lindsey's "Systems Approach to Marriage and Family Therapy" course, we were asked to reflect on what it means to regulate emotions and the benefits of doing so to help with expressing empathy while in session with a client. My classmate, Gaby, made the comment that this exercise was not designed for "us," meaning the students of Color. Without her even needing to explain her thought process, I knew immediately why she was feeling that way. As Lindsey walked up to our group to check in on us, Gaby shared this thought. It was apparent that Lindsey was not quite sure how to take this comment, but remained curious. I chimed in and explained that people of Color are experts at emotional regulation. We learn the importance of the skill as children. Lindsey still seemed uncertain about the point we were trying to make and asked us to hold our thoughts on the subject until the class reconvened as a whole after the group exercise so that all could hear and take part in the conversation.

Once the class was together in its entirety again, she asked Gaby and I to share the thoughts and comments with the class that we had just shared with her. I explained that as people of Color, it was important for us to learn emotional regulation as children for safety purposes. This extends to all marginalized communities as well. Gaby explained that in certain situations, it could be harmful for a therapist of Color to empathize with a White client if they do not hold that individual accountable for their thoughts or actions. Showing sympathy for a client, staying curious, and respecting their lived experience can still be accomplished without losing yourself as the therapist. The ways in which we bring our experiences in the broader social context into this unique role are complex, and what became clear as we continued to talk was the need to address these questions from each person's social location and position of power instead of a "one size fits all."

A couple of weeks after this class discussion, Lindsey reached out to Gaby and me for a meeting to further discuss our perspectives on the topic and to better understand where we were coming from. This really was a growing moment for all three of us. Gaby and I were able to share an even more nuanced perspective from our lens with Lindsey, and Lindsey demonstrated the humanism of being both a therapist and a professor by not challenging our lived experiences, but instead genuinely wanting to understand where we were coming from. She allowed us to impact her and shift her thinking, while simultaneously teaching Gaby and I what it looks like to humble oneself and to stay curious.

6   Gaby

There is so much conversation happening around identity, especially on college campuses. Who we are and how we identify is both deeply personal and for many of us political. I identify as an Afro-Latina, my mom is Dominican, and my father is Puerto Rican. I am a first-generation college student, and first to be working toward a master's degree. My husband and I have been married for 8 years and have a 4-year-old and 2-year-old. The shift from being a married couple to parents has been both terrifying and incredibly rewarding. As an interracial couple we have had to be very intentional in our marriage and how we parent. A lot of our life experiences are different from each other's, and there are times when my husband, who is white, does not show up to situations in ways that I would like. He has not ever needed to think about identity in the ways that I (or in the future, our biracial children) have. It takes many open and vulnerable conversations for my view to be seen. This can be hard on a marriage.

Regardless of where people are in their anti-racist work, hard conversations must be had, and what makes them so hard is what these truths mean about our positions in the world. It is less about reaching the highest level of understanding and more about being a constant learner and evaluator of the systems around us. Building a life with someone and raising children together requires so much empathy and self-reflection. I have had to learn to empathize with my own experiences, to have empathy through the learning curves of life, and for my children who both need empathy to be modeled. My children have shown me that there is a full range of humanity, and they are teaching me patience, compassion, and the importance of inner child work.

My first semester in my MFT program, there were several conversations that challenged me and have been topics that I think about often. Our professor, Lindsey, would assign readings and then in class we would have small group discussions that then would open to the whole class. One reading was about emotional regulation as a therapist and was written by several women of color. We were asked to imagine being in different marginalized communities outside of our own real identities, and to think through how we might manage working with clients who challenge those identities. The prompt felt to me like it implicitly assumed that therapists come from a position of power. While this is often true in some regards (therapists have graduate degrees, etc.), this would have worked better if framed to identify one's actual social locations and positions of social power first. As I shared these thoughts, Lindsey heard us and brought the conversation back to the whole class. Personally, I appreciated having a whole class discussion about it – it felt like equity. Having a classroom where students can respectfully give feedback, especially for a white teacher who is talking about marginalized groups, is all the difference between oppressive environments and one that is learning and growing together.

The second conversation that came up in class was around being empathetic toward people who come from very different lived experiences. In theory that sounds solid. It also sounds like it was centered around a white heteronormative hypothetical therapist. I thought, "What would that look like for me? What am I the most nervous about?" The first thing that popped into my mind was a white man who comes into session and dumps all his racist ideas about different groups in my lap. In this hypothetical, he is polite and then angry if challenged, and entitled in the sense that he sees me and feels I should agree with whatever stereotypes he believes about people of color he has encountered. There is a long history centered around women of color and their role as caretakers.

Having this in mind, all I could think of was "How could I be empathetic toward a racist that believes it is my role to accommodate their every thought?" To that I said "HELL NO." I knew this was not what Lindsey was implying, and at the same time it felt like something she was not aware of as being ever-present for people like me. These stereotypes are very much alive and show up in various ways. Therefore, it is so important that anti-racist work and education around critical race theory happen alongside all course work and disciplines. Racism is happening all the time everywhere and facing it head-on is the only way to see how it is showing up in classrooms. Both of these conversations are for me a testament to the impact classrooms have on their students, outside of the course content. The conversations offered all of us a moment of pause to evaluate what was coming up for some of us and what was not for others. I will admit that initially my "hell no" did not come across to me as an emotional response. It was a blockade to protect myself, and had I not had a professor who wanted to know my experiences, I would not have become aware of my own biases around what I had to learn about conversations like these.

Our program has a students of color group called PLUS (PLU Students of Color). I went to this group after these interactions, feeling like I needed a space where I did not have to explain myself. I wanted to talk to other women of color about what empathy means in therapy when coming up against a client who is saying or doing things that affect us personally. What I found was a huge spectrum of thought around what empathy means when you are a marginalized person. I had to dissect empathy for myself; there is a vulnerability when we have empathy for others. It is not the difference between a therapist who has a client who has a different view about something. It is about a therapist who has a client who does not see them as a human being. That distinction between "we don't agree" and "you question my personhood" is what makes this empathy piece so challenging.

This is not the kind of topic that has resolution. But I did have a realization that I have been empathetic in situations that felt like my hypothetical. I can be empathetic without validating. I can feel empathy about the path that may have impacted someone in a way that makes them believe racist rhetoric. But I do not need to validate those thoughts. It is a delicate dance of protecting myself from emotional harm and feeling like I am the best person to handle those moments. Just to be clear, these thoughts are my own, and my opinions about these hypotheticals and the role of empathy is ever-changing. I have gone from "hell no" to "maybe." The "maybe" depends on the context and the person's level of awareness.

After this class discussion, Lindsey asked Nicki and me to have a conversation about what came up in class. I went into the meeting a bit skeptical and unsure, but what unfolded allowed the three of us to have an impactful conversation stemming from Lindsey's genuine desire to understand where we were coming from. She was willing to listen without any defensiveness, and because of that, it was a powerful exchange. Instead of putting herself in our shoes (as was the assignment in class), she just believed us. Academia places so much importance on titles, as opposed to seeing places of learning as intertwined and dependent on the transfer of information from teacher to students and students to teacher. Lindsey opening our comments to the class and then taking some time to think about it and wanting more clarity in our second conversation honored this fluid way of learning and acquiring knowledge. I felt heard and more importantly I felt like I was a holder of important knowledge too, which was empowering.

7 Conclusion

There are two themes the three of us have continued to circle back to as our conversations around this topic keep unfolding. The first is that change happens in relationships with one another. I (LN) am changed in ways I could not be otherwise through the impact of my students and their vulnerability and care for me. No textbook, no conference, no anti-bias training impacts me the way those relationships do. Our relationships give us a framework for learning and growing, as Gaby said, in a multi-directional way. The second is that nuance matters. We do not have many examples of nuanced, productive, cross-racial conversations happening today. That needs to shift, and the responsibility lies first with white folks in listening and believing the experiences of people of Color. When I listened to Nicki and Gaby, my initial fears of "what if we don't agree on this?" quickly dissipated. As we talked through things – what empathy means to each of us, how we have experienced empathy differently, our fears around empathy, and how our different identities impact what is expected of us around empathy – we were able to connect and empathize with one another, even though our lived experiences were different. Through the gifts of relationships and nuanced conversations, we hope others – educators and students alike – can experience the transforming personal, professional, and political changes that move us all toward better caring for each other.

References

Allan, R., & Singh Poulsen, S. (Eds.). (2017). *Creating cultural safety in couple and family therapy supervision and training.* Springer.

Eppler, C. (2021). Dismantling whiteness to direct a just couples and family therapy program: Experiences of a white program director. In K. Quek & A. Hsieh (Eds.), *Intersectionality in family therapy leadership: Professional power, personal identities* (pp. 81–92). Springer.

Garcia, M., Kosutic, I., & McDowell, T. (2015). Peace on earth/war at home: The role of emotion regulation in social justice work. *Journal of Feminist Family Therapy, 27,* 1–20.

Hardy, K. (Ed.). (2022). *The enduring, invisible, and ubiquitous centrality of whiteness.* W.W. Norton & Co.

Hardy, K., & Bobes, T. (Eds.). (2016). *Culturally sensitive supervision and training: Diverse perspectives and practical applications.* Routledge.

Hardy, K., & McGoldrick, M. (2019). Re-visioning family therapy training. In M. McGoldrick & K. Hardy (Eds.), *Re-visioning family therapy: Addressing diversity in clinical practice* (pp. 477–495). Guilford.

Kendall, M. (2020). *Hood feminism: Notes from the women that a movement forgot.* Penguin Random House.

McDowell, T., & Shelton, D. (2002). Valuing ideas of social justice in MFT curricula. *Contemporary Family Therapy, 24*(2), 313–331.

McGoldrick, M., Almeida, R., Garcia Preto, N., Bibb, A., Sutton, C., Hudak, J., & Moore Hines, P. (1999). Efforts to incorporate social justice perspectives into a family therapy training program. *Journal of Marital and Family Therapy, 25*(2), 191–209. https://doi.org/10.1111/j.1752-0606.1999.tb01122.x

Price, T. A. (2015). *The black therapist-white client counseling dyad: The relationship between black racial identity and countertransference.* Lehigh University, Counseling Psychology Department Theses and Dissertations, pp. 1–154. http://preserve.lehigh.edu/etd/2769

Pugh, C. (Podcast host). (2020). *There is no such thing as a white ally.* Retrieved from ♃There Is No Such Thing as a 'White Ally' — "TNSWA" Part I. | by Catherine Pugh, Esq. | CIVIS ROMANUS | Medium

Quek, K. M., & Hsieh, A. L. (Eds.). (2021). *Intersectionality in family therapy leadership: Professional power, personal identities.* Springer.

Tatum, B. D. (2017). *Why are all the black kids sitting together in the cafeteria? And other conversations about race.* Basic Books.

Woodson, J. (2018). *The day you begin.* Nancy Paulson Books.

"We've Got This": Unburdening the Pressure of Identity Through Co-teaching

Justine D'Arrigo and Jessica ChenFeng

In this chapter we share about our experience of co-teaching a socio-cultural diversity course from different personal identity perspectives of race, gender, and sexuality. We discuss the ways in which having various representations of identities in the classroom allowed us to approach charged topics, like systems of power and oppression, from a relational perspective, which can be difficult to do when teaching alone. The opportunity we had in this co-teaching relationship was made possible by the cultivation of a deep friendship outside our roles as professors. We offer a bit about how our friendship evolved while navigating mixed-identities and discuss how this invited us into relational intentionality in ways we had not necessarily experienced so explicitly in friendships before. Part of what made this friendship possible and so valuable to our co-teaching of this course was a clear commitment we both held to examining and understanding the real effects of how operations of power and oppression related to our differing identities, and then how this worked to organize and shape the way we engaged relationally. This awareness, in part, produced our decision to teach together, knowing full well that university systems often try to use diversity and representation as a rationale to slate faculty of color into teaching diversity-related courses without acknowledging or considering the larger structural risks for these faculty.

For us, the value of this experience is rooted in the opportunity we had to transform course content into a lived experience, an experience where students were able to witness the ways in which learning about and understanding issues of race, power, and privilege actually shape and inform the ways relationships are

J. D'Arrigo (✉)
California State University, San Bernardino, CA, USA
e-mail: justine.darrigopatrick@csusb.edu

J. ChenFeng
Fuller Theological Seminary, Pasadena, CA, USA

© American Family Therapy Academy (AFTA) 2023
L. A. Nice, C. Eppler (eds.), *Social Justice and Systemic Family Therapy Training*,
AFTA SpringerBriefs in Family Therapy, https://doi.org/10.1007/978-3-031-29930-8_2

coordinated. In this case, how we – their professors – from different racial experiences, gender experiences, cultural experiences, etc., showed up in relationship together, taking responsibility for their places of privilege, and how we step into accountability with one another for the places where structural and systemic oppression show up differently.

1 Background Considerations

Historically, diversity courses were primarily taught from a multicultural framework that often neglected attending to systemic practices of power and oppression (Ortiz & Jani, 2010). The multicultural framework encouraged professors, both faculty of color and white faculty, to teach from a model that reduced diversity to racial and ethnic group differences based on varying cultural values, norms, and practices (Polk et al., 2021). Some of the consequences of this framework are that it can end up solidifying stereotypes and cultural caricatures, overemphasizing between-group differences and minimizing variability and within-group differences. Overall, it can have the unintended effect of rendering racial and ethnic communities as monolithic groups with essentialized qualities (Abrams & Moio, 2009). In this context, systemic oppression, structural inequity and the complex power relations that construct society in specific and intentional ways get overlooked (Ortiz & Jani, 2010). This allows these courses to be seen as apolitical, positioning course content as anthropological fact and instructors simply as objective distributors of cultural information. The problem with this is that it often obscures the ways in which these courses, particularly when taught by white faculty members, work to reify colorblind ideologies that perpetuate and maintain white supremacy in the field and the academy (Abrams & Moio, 2009; Ortiz & Jani, 2010; Polk et al., 2021).

In the recent decade, there has been a growing emphasis on diversifying the academy and increasing representation among program faculty, while also shifting the focus and emphasis away from multiculturalism in these courses to a more power attentive perspective of social justice. The convergence of these trends has meant that minoritized professors often become the ones responsible for teaching these courses that are now seen as more "politically liberal" with an agenda to disrupt deeply held American Values (Ruby, 2022). As faculty of color are tasked with the work of deconstructing white supremacy and teaching about the historical foundations of colonialism, they become saddled with a heavy burden as white students can be explicitly resistant to these themes (Vianden, 2018). This often contributes to an unfavorable teaching environment for minoritized faculty, and at times can be actively hostile for them. This is also part of what influenced us in choosing to coteach this course together, which we expand on in the following text.

2 Overview of Our Approach

When we were doctoral students, we had the opportunity to teach a course on gender, race, and class. Instead of teaching our own sections, we decided to combine our students so that we could co-teach. I am not sure we had the research, theory, and language to explain why this was our preference, but we had a sense that a course like this would be less difficult to teach in partnership with two instructors with different intersectional identities. What we describe here as our "approach" is not a model, but the experience we had and our reflections around it. We are not suggesting that it is the best or right way; rather, it is what we tried and it ended up being powerfully meaningful to us and our students.

Foundational to how we approached co-teaching was centering our relationship and the power that relationships have to catalyze change and growth. Gender, race, and class (social context) are not merely topics; they are connected to individuals' and communities' identities and all of it informs and shapes how we engage with one another in relationship. To us, there is little meaning without understanding how social context organizes relationships. Thus, we sought to "go public with our relationship," that is, making our relational process known to the students, a process that was going to be explicit about our social contextual selves. Along the way, we invited students to be witness to how the concepts of gender, race, and class informed our decisions about teaching and our process of collaborative negotiation.

With relationship at the core, our co-teaching then had two main areas of focus: how we navigated our co-teaching dynamics, and what we hoped students would learn through witnessing and engaging in the relational process with us. In considering our co-teaching dynamics, we wanted to make sure that we regularly attended to our working relationship, attuned to the other person's minoritized identities, and used our voice of privilege whenever possible. Both of us have minoritized and privileged parts of our identity, some more visible (like racial identity) and others less visible (social class, sexual orientation, etc.). Because of our friendship, we knew about each other's lived experiences around our minoritized identities so we could have intentional conversations about how we would navigate these in class. For example, I (Jessica) knew and trusted that Justine had witnessed and cared about the racist experiences I have had as an Asian American. So during class time, if we were addressing the experiences of people/women of color and encountered students' micro-aggressive or dismissive comments, I knew that Justine was attuning to me and the content such that they could step into that space and use their voice as a white person. This is a different experience from most typical diversity course structures taught by a person of color. When white students are activated or upset about conversations regarding race, it is stressful and sometimes traumatic for a professor of color to address, let alone challenge, the student. In co-teaching, we wanted to model to students that our working relationship was valuable to us and to use our privilege with accountability and humility.

I (Justine) was able to lean on the relational foundation that Jessica and I had cultivated in moments where students' hetero privilege showed up in subtle yet impactful ways, and even times when more direct expressions of homophobia were enacted by students. These moments, while uncomfortable, were less distressing for me in the context of co-teaching than when teaching alone. Jessica was aware of, concerned for, and attentive to the emotional impact of these moments for me and was willing to use her voice as a cis-hetero professor to invite students into reflection about the impact of their words and beliefs. This dynamic produced an opportunity to teach from a more vulnerable place, knowing that we always held care and protection of one another at the center.

What we hoped students would learn through witnessing and engaging with us is what it could look like to consider our privileged identities and how they can support and uphold people and relationships. This is counter to what is often felt in regard to the idea of having privilege: shame, discomfort, paralysis about what to do with privilege. We understand some of this shame to be related to the lack of relational depth that we share with those who have minoritized identities. In our relationship, we have wrestled and sought to be present with one another in all parts of our identities, particularly with minoritization. In sitting with one another, we learned how to support each other and when, or if, to speak up for the other.

We also hoped for students to witness the unease and tension of difficult conversations about social context and to develop the stamina required to sit in and navigate through such tension. It is one thing to sit and be present with clients' emotional distress; it is another type of emotional capacity, which requires developing, to sit with our own internal discomfort around self-identity and relational tension. Our experience is that unless we have had the gift of engaging at these depths in personal relationships, it is nearly impossible to teach and model to students, particularly developing therapists, how to do the same.

3   Our Experience: Activism Through Relationship

In this section, we share our co-teaching experience in more depth. We attempt to address the question around how we came to engage in activism through relationship. How is it that we developed a relationship of trust for anti-racist practice, privilege, and accountability work?

3.1   Early Connection: Who We Are, Our Intersections of Identity, and How We Found Friendship with One Another

It is hard to say exactly who we are, both because we are not now who we were then, and in the years to come, we will not be who we are today. However, we think there is a common thread between the two of us as well as between the multiple iterations of ourselves over the years, and that thread is the importance of tending to relationships. This quickly became a place of common ground between the two of us when we met in our doctoral program at Loma Linda University. Although we had this place of shared values, I would also say that at first, for me (Justine), there was some self-protection and hesitancy I felt toward entering into relationship with Jessica, not because of anything Jessica had said or done to make the relationship feel unsafe but purely because one of our first connections was around our shared faith. At the time, I identified as a lesbian woman, but was not out publicly to family or within school and work contexts. When Jessica shared with me that she had gone to Fuller Theological Seminary and was a practicing Christian, this part of her identity made me wary, and even though I had a shared Christian background, my painful experiences in the church had led me to move away from those communities and relationships. I was not interested at the time in having to justify or explain the validity of my sexuality, nor was I interested in another relationship with someone who professed to care for me but could not condone my "lifestyle." It is important to note, there is nothing Jessica ever said that was directly diminishing of my sexuality, but it was the very fact that she carried the identity of being a Christian that made me assume all of these things might be at play for her.

The other reality was that I enjoyed her very much. I found her to be one of my cohort mates that I connected very well with and over time, we grew closer and started to dialogue about some of these tensions in our identities. I think part of this evolution for me was the way Jessica remained curious about and engaged with me. Jessica was incredibly respectful and honoring of my initial hesitance. She also was not deterred by my hesitance, and gently persisted in her interest in being my friend. The effect this had was that my hesitance and reservations began to recede, and my friendship with her grew in ways that profoundly impacted me and became restorative in places where there had been harm done as a result of homophobia in the church and broader culture. I often tell people that Jessica, at that time, created a bridge for me to reconnect with my treasured spirituality, although in a new way than before.

What I (Jessica) remember about our early connections is that I thought Justine was down-to-earth, authentic, and not afraid of difficult conversations. At that point in my life, I had not yet developed meaningful cross-racial friendships that could talk about race; this meant that I had never really felt known by a non-Asian friend. I did not know how to articulate my own racialized experiences, nor had I ever encountered a non-Asian person being interested in me or my people's racial realities. It was a different experience with Justine. They were genuinely curious about my experiences as a Taiwanese American woman. When they noticed me being treated differently (going out to eat as a group and I was the only non-white peer), they expressed anger, validated my experience, and were able to speak to racism directly. I did not feel the need to protect any white fragility or sugarcoat my reality so as to shield them from feeling discomfort; this was something I was used to doing in most other parts of my life. I will address this more later, but seeing Justine stay engaged in understanding their whiteness and caring about my racialized experiences gave me the impression that this was not just going to be a friendship to maintain. It could maybe be a friendship where I could be my authentic self and we could share life with one another.

3.2   Trust Building

Mutual trust is critical for each of us to feel known, be willing to be known, and genuinely want to know the other. It meant the world to me (Jessica) that a white friend was starting to really get my experiences as an Asian American woman in the world. It was disorienting for me because I rarely had the chance to reflect out loud about Asian American racism, invisibility, and my own experiences with model minority and honorary white stereotypes. Oftentimes, Justine would pick up on some part of my own internalized racism and validate an experience for me before I could even articulate it for myself. This was powerfully healing for me – that a white friend would care so much, do their own ongoing work, such that I felt truly seen. This went beyond our friendship in that I saw and knew that Justine was regularly involved in learning more about and advocating on behalf of issues of equity and justice. I experienced them as someone with deep integrity – accountable to themselves, to others, and to their values.

I grew up in a conservative Asian American Christian context where there were strong beliefs and sentiments about sexual orientation. These were largely unexamined for much of my life because there was little in my context to challenge these beliefs and offer other perspectives. While it had been a few years of me deconstructing these beliefs, it was not until I met Justine that I came to see the depth and harm of my homophobia and binary mindsets. Because I was so acutely aware of my experience in the world as an Asian American woman (my minoritized identities), it was a challenge to start navigating my privilege as a Christian heterosexual cisgender person. As we connected and I heard more about Justine's painful experiences with the Christian church, I knew that I could not keep going on with my unexamined beliefs. I was compelled to do some real excavation because Justine mattered to me, I believed that God loved them, and it was important to me that I lived with congruence in faith and life. Over the coming months and years, I read books, articles, and went to workshops and conferences that challenged and facilitated this journey. I believe that God was expanding my mind and heart and I will forever be grateful that my friendship with Justine led me to encounter such healing, transformation, and depth of spiritual growth.

When I (Justine) met Jessica, I had very little practice with sharing about my sexuality openly at all, let alone with someone who I knew who identified as cis, hetero, and Christian, identities I came to know as threatening. However, the friendship we began cultivating quickly became one of the safest relational spaces in my life at that time, aside from my partner. Jessica's interest and curiosity about my experiences seemed to emanate from a genuinely caring relational posture of humility and concern rather than nosiness or exploitation, both of which I was very familiar with from earlier life experiences. Her honest care and interest put me at ease in a way that was rare for me to experience, particularly with someone who identified as a Christian. My experience of Jessica at this time was that she was interested in my experience not to correct or change me by being a loving "witness" but as a way to examine and possibly change her own heart. I had not had a relational encounter with a hetero cisgender Christian before where there seemed to be such willingness to learn from me and my experiences in a way that would produce shifts, changes, and alterations in their own beliefs. This was compelling for me, and as a result deeply affected me in ways that were restorative and healing. I also admired and respected that Jessica was a friend that took on such accountability for doing her own work. She sought out conversations with others, read articles and books, and would choose to step into humble conversation with me about how her heart and beliefs were being challenged and expanded, even as unanswered questions lingered. Jessica was always attentive and accountable to places where she may have been operating from her heteronormative privilege and would come to me when she thought she may have said something that could have the potential to leave me feeling tender. I remember a time when she had made a comment about marriage, and at the time I remember mentioning how I did not have that same choice that she had, and I could tell it created a moment of pause for her. Rather than feeling bad, Jessica acknowledged that with me in the moment, and later came back to the conversation to share with me about the ways she was seeing how her heteronormative lens was taken for granted in so many subtle ways and how she was beginning to unpack that. This created even more trust between us, and provided safety for me knowing I did not have to raise things or bring them to her attention, because I knew that she was doing the work to see them on her own and then reflect with me.

Aside from my own queerness, so many of my earlier life experiences situated me to hold a deep place of understanding of what it meant and felt like to be othered. So, as I got to know Jessica, there was a sense of understanding, in part, of her experiences of having to navigate the many damaging effects attached to the "model minority" moniker as well as more blatant racism as a result of her visible Taiwanese American identity. However, being white, I knew very well how deeply white supremacy had trained me to not see many of the places where I lived with privilege. Because of this, I knew I had to be committed to always doing my best to hold this in view and to inspect the ways this showed up in our friendship, as well as our teaching relationship. I often thought I had a good grasp on my awareness of how this happened, though there were many times when I saw how my privilege as a white person really shaped the way I felt comfortable to use my voice with students and others and assume no consequence for it, when that same privilege was not often the same kind of fail-safe for Jessica.

3.3 Acceptance of Internal Struggles

When it comes to developing an honest, mutually supportive relationship, I (Jessica) believe that it is our fear of rejection, remaining unknown, and also being truly known that prevents us from moving toward connection. I can think back to the many internal struggles I had throughout the course of our friendship. Even now, I have a sense that there are many layers of my own racialized identity that I have yet to uncover. I had never talked with anyone about the weight of racism that I carry with me all the time – not even to myself. I experience this to be largely self-protective and a form of racial resilience I have had to build in order to keep going.

It felt scary to explore these inner dynamics with Justine, for them to make reflections back to me about my identity, and to start feeling vulnerable and known in these parts of myself. I could not hide behind the complexities of my model minority identity with this white friend.

I also struggled with not wanting my own journey as a Christian deconstructing homophobia to be hurtful for Justine and wondered to what degree I share about that process with them. I knew they had been so hurt by the Christian church and I did not want to contribute to that pain. I felt some sort of responsibility, personally and communally, as someone who was part of the Christian community to acknowledge and take personal ownership of the deep hurt that Christians have inflicted on the queer community. Though it was uncomfortable, I knew I needed to move toward the discomfort of recognizing that it was the sort of homophobia and fundamentalist ideology I grew up with that forced beloved siblings like Justine out of the church. In accepting my own internal struggles, I felt more integrated with myself and the history of which I was a part.

There were struggles for me (Justine) around what it meant to navigate my whiteness and privilege in the context of relationship with Jessica without feeling like that invalidated any place of tenderness I held around my identity as a queer person, and the harm I had experienced at the hands of Christian cisgender hetero folks. I held a lot of anger that was rooted in such deep pain and I sometimes felt unsure of how to speak to this in congruent and honest ways with Jessica. I worried it would be too harsh or even antagonistic toward a part of her identity that she held so dear. I was also very new to speaking about my queerness, and at the time, there were many things I had yet to understand about what being queer meant for me. So much of what I was navigating then was about my sexuality, but I was also internally exploring so many other complexities – things I had not shared or even looked at closely for myself. I felt like the church in many ways was responsible for what felt like my late blooming, and my resentment was palpable. I took care with how to communicate about this because I wanted to protect Jessica, and did not want what felt like my messy process to create painful places for her in return. Jessica, however, often invited my raw feelings forward, and heard them, held them, and witnessed them in gracious and compassionate ways. These conversations could often feel quite vulnerable, but because we held such tremendous space for gentleness, grace, and trust in one another, we were able to sit in the tension of these often unknown and uncharted relational territories. So much of this was made possible by holding deep care and respect at the center of our friendship.

4   How Our Experience Informed Co-teaching

As we share our co-teaching experience, we want to remind readers that this is not a model or any best/right way to co-teach. Our co-teaching experience was very much an extension of our friendship's journey. In this section, we want to share how our choiceful negotiations shaped our teaching together, as well as specific experiences that impacted the way we continue to think about mixed-identity friend-ship and co-teaching.

One of the things that we were very clear about in our co-teaching process is that we wanted to be transparent with students about what our teaching process was. This meant that we were intentional about exposing the ways identity shaped our choices in how to facilitate the overall course as well as each week's lessons and activities. In practice this often looked like sharing with the class the kinds of con-versations we had with one another in preparation for the day's lecture, specifically sharing about how each one of us reflected on how our differing identities informed or might have informed how we were each thinking about it. In many ways we would "go public" with our planning process and would invite students to offer their thoughts and reflections about what we were sharing. This created a space where students were also able to share thoughts and ideas about the facilitation of class that were informed by their various identities. At times, we invited them to help decide how we might proceed in class, at other times we made the decision, but always shared the background details of how we arrived at the decision. This was important to us because the material we were teaching about – diversity, equity, and justice – mattered a lot, but it did not matter if they did not learn how it shaped the ways we navigate the influence of interpersonal dynamics. We wanted what we were teaching to make a real-time relational difference. We did not just want to teach concepts, we wanted to create a container for safe and transformative experiences.

One formative experience we had together happened outside of the classroom and outside of any conversation or planning session for class. At some point before or during the quarter we were co-teaching, we were walking back to our cars together and had to cross the street on a crosswalk. The way I (Jessica) remember it is that when it was safe to cross, I hurriedly walked across the street while Justine (in my opinion) seemed to take their time. My (Justine's) memory of these details is a bit different, and it seemed we were waiting at the crosswalk for a minute or so and the cars were not stopping for us. So I stepped into the crosswalk, while Jessica appeared to be hanging back, wanting to wait for the cars to yield to us. I remember saying something like, "We have the right of way Jess, come on, they have to stop for us." Now, setting aside the details of exactly how it transpired, we both noticed a difference in how we approached something as simple as a crosswalk. In debrief-ing with one another, we realized that something as seemingly mundane as crossing the street was a racialized experience. I (Jessica) felt that if I appeared to take my time and space, drivers would see me, an Asian American woman, and attribute all kinds of negative thoughts and assumptions about my race. "Look at that slow inconsiderate Asian woman;" "Asian people are so _____." My (Justine's) reflec-tions were along the lines of "It's our right of way as pedestrians!" This seemed to reflect my taken-for-granted white privilege and the differing racialized socializa-tion I experienced growing up, which taught me that I had rights and could take up space in a way that I did not need to be apologetic for. Though a bit humorous, this interaction gave us both increased insight into how much our identities shape choices, behaviors, thoughts, and relational stress in every facet of our daily living.

We wanted to make it exceptionally clear for our students that we actively attuned to, and navigated with one another, the varied ways that power and identity organizes relationships and relational dynamics. This became an explicit conversation in our class when we facilitated a fishbowl activity around the social construction of race. Part of this lesson was to unpack the construct of race and deconstruct the belief that race is a biological reality. Part of what we had students do was to sit with other students in the class whom they believed they shared the most genetic similarity. As predicted, many of the students sat with other students that outwardly appeared to share similar ethnic and racial identities. While we took care to deconstruct the idea of race with our class, we were also intentional to name the real effects of race on lived experience, even if it was a social construct. As part of this activity we wanted each racial grouping of students to discuss some of the stereotypes and assumptions that they felt were often made about groups and people who looked the way they did, and some of the challenges or experiences this created for them in their lives. We wanted this to be a witnessing activity with one group at a time sitting in the center of the circle and having a conversation with one another about this.

The part of this activity that really brought in discussions of power and identity was when it came time to negotiate the question of which group should share first. Jessica and I discussed with the class some of the thoughts and conversations we had. We shared that we had thought through multiple ways of possibly doing this portion of the activity and our concerns about each of the possibilities. On the one hand, we thought it might be appropriate to have the group of white students share first, and that in some way choosing this may account for power in a way that it would ask them to be vulnerable with the group first. The concern about having them go first was that white people are often the ones noticed and heard from first, so would this potentially reify a position of power for white students? If a group of students of color go first, would this also support more equity in the room by allow-ing their voices to be centered and heard first, or did asking them to go first burden them with more vulnerability? We shared that we had not come to a conclusion about what was best, and invited their input and feedback, but we were also trans-parent with them that no matter how we decided to move forward as a class, the learning was in asking these questions. Recognizing and accounting for the ways we arrive at particular decisions, and the potential consequences of those decisions, should always be a part of how those decisions get made, even if there are no clear answers or perfect solutions.

5 Research-Based Reflections and Encouragements for Colleagues

We know from anecdotal experiences of minoritized faculty, as well as the literature on this topic, that co-teaching across identities is supported. The literature is clear about the negative impact for faculty of color in bearing the burden of teaching diversity related courses on their own, particularly with a high percentage of white students in the room, which is often the case for most graduate couple and family therapy programs. For faculty of color, teaching white students about their privilege and whiteness often results in poor teacher course evaluations (Boatright-Horowitz & Soeung, 2009), and more critical ratings on teacher evaluations than white teachers (Williams & Evans-Winters, 2005). As teachers of color, Puchner and Roseboro (2011) talk about addressing this challenge by adopting what they call "A pedagogy of purposeful compromise." They suggest that in order to begin conversations about white privilege with white students they must begin by privileging whiteness and the experiences of white students instead of starting out with visibilizing the experiences of students of color. This requires faculty of color to background their own marginalized experiences, which also backgrounds the experiences of students of color in the courses as well. While adaptive, we see this as reflective of the lasting effects of colonization within academia, and that "pacifying white students is done at the cost of critical learning and silencing faculty and students of color" (McDowell & Hernandez, 2010).

Additional challenges faculty of color face include larger structural and systemic constraints at the university level. Ahmed (2008) noted university and anti-racist policy as a prominent barrier in effectively being able to teach from a critical perspective, drawing attention to the reality that although some universities promote acknowledgment of diversity and equity, they are often vague in their position statements. This creates conflicting messages about the extent to which "critical perspectives" should be incorporated into university curriculum (Ahmed, 2008), leaving faculty of color vulnerable to being questioned for taking bold and counter cultural stands. Again, we believe that co-teaching with mixed identity faculty has the potential to distribute this kind of burden more equitably so that the weight is not entirely placed on one professor.

These kinds of co-teaching relationships are particularly important as teachers of color continue to be asked and expected to bear the burden of responsibility for making power visible, confronting white supremacy, and illuminating the various effects these have on client experience and the field of therapy. Universities often try to couch these course assignments within the narrative of representation and inclusion, yet willfully ignore the personal and professional vulnerabilities this exposes faculty of color to, as classroom ratings directly impact evaluation for tenure and promotion. Overlooking these consequences reinforces structural racism. To counteract this, or to further expose the double standard in teaching evaluations, white professors should be stepping in alongside faculty of color in ways that do not contribute to them being the sole target of white students' fragility (Pewewardy, 2004).

What we have briefly outlined here certainly supports co-teaching efforts in these contexts whenever possible to do so. It was not until some time after that we were able to see the significance of this decision, and the ways in which it stood against the relational and systemic harm often perpetuated against minoritized faculty left to teach these courses on their own.

Our experience is one example of co-teaching and we certainly do not presume to have implications solely based on our experience and co-teaching relationship.

We do, however, have encouragements for our educator colleagues. Because a foundational value we hold is that "We teach who we are" (Palmer, 2017), these are our encouragements to you.

5.1 Consider Co-Teaching with Mixed-Identity Colleagues (Colleague-of-Color with White Colleague, Different Gender Identities, Sexual Orientations, Religious/Spiritual Background, etc.)

In a field such as family therapy where isomorphic processes exist across many relational levels (supervisor/educator to supervisee/student to client), we believe that mixed-identity co-teachers offer an ideal teaching dynamic. Because race is a fundamental stratifier in our society, having an educator of color and a white educator is not only valuable but perhaps even necessary for establishing psychological safety for both students and faculty.

5.2 Have Meta-Conversations About the Co-teaching Relationship

Having diversity with the co-teachers is not simply a box to check off. It is the starting piece of an enriching teaching and learning environment. Because of the different social locations of the co-teachers, it is important for them to be in conversation about their co-teaching dynamics inside and outside of the classroom. This is similar to what therapists often encourage couples to do; they promote meta-conversation about the relationship, rather than simply talk about what each person wants to do, eat, etc. The content of the course will be figured out, but more critical is the relational dynamics between the co-teachers, exploring how power and marginalization plays out in their interactions, and what it looks like to allow these awarenesses to be part of the teaching experience.

5.3 Allow What Matters to Your Colleague to Matter to You

Some of the challenges of teaching in the current climate is that it is too easy to put someone else into the category of "the other." The moment we sense that someone has a different opinion, point-of-view, political ideology, educational background, etc., we hold them at arm's length, often because of the fear or judgment we have. When co-teachers, with all their differences, can come together not only to talk about their separate identities, but to really model caring for each other's communities, this is the most powerful influence on witnessing students.

We value the time readers have spent engaging with our reflections about our co-teaching experience. We hope that it encourages and challenges you to consider the complexities of faculty identities as they intersect with teaching diversity courses.

References

Abrams, L. S., & Moio, J. A. (2009). Critical race theory and the cultural competence dilemma in social work education. *Journal of Social Work Education, 45*(2), 254–261.

Ahmed, B. (2008). Teaching critical psychology of 'race' issues: Problems in promoting anti-racist practice. *Journal of Community & Applied Social Psychology, 18*, 54–67.

Boatright-Horowitz, S. L., & Soeung, S. (2009). Teaching white privilege to white students can mean saying good-bye to positive student evaluations. *American Psychologist, 64*(6), 574–575. https://doi.org/10.1037/a0016593

McDowell, T., & Hernandez, P. (2010). Decolonizing academia: Intersectionality, participation, and accountability in family therapy and counseling. *Journal of Feminist Family Therapy, 22*(2), 93–111. https://doi.org/10.1080/08952831003787834

Ortiz, L., & Jani, J. (2010). Critical race theory: A transformational model for teaching diversity. *Journal of Social Work Education, 46*(2), 175–193.

Palmer, P. J. (2017). *The courage to teach: Exploring the inner landscape of a teacher's life.* Jossey-Bass.

Pewewardy, N. (2004). The political is personal: The essential obligation of white feminist family therapists to deconstruct white privilege. *Journal of Feminist Family Therapy, 16*(1), 53–67. https://doi.org/10.1300/J086v16n01_05

Polk, S. A., Vazquez, N., Kim, M. E., & Green, Y. R. (2021). Moving from multiculturalism to critical race theory within a school of social work: Dismantling white supremacy as an organizing strategy. *Advances in Social Work, 21*(2), 876–897. https://doi.org/10.18060/24472

Puchner, L., & Roseboro, D. L. (2011). Speaking of whiteness: Compromise as a purposeful pedagogical strategy toward white students' learning about race. *Teaching in Higher Education, 16*(4), 377–387. https://doi.org/10.1080/13562517.2010.546528

Ruby, T. F. (2022). The American dream, colorblind ideology, and nationalism: Teaching diversity courses as a woman faculty of color. *Journal of Women and Gender in Higher Education, 15*(2), 201–219. https://doi.org/10.1080/26379112.2022.2068023

Vianden, J. (2018). "In all honesty, you don't learn much": White college men's perceptions of diversity courses and instructors. *International Journal of Teaching and Learning in Higher Education, 30*(3), 465–476.

Williams, D. G., & Evans-Winters, V. (2005). The burden of teaching teachers: Memoirs of race discourse in teacher education. *The Urban Review, 37*(3), 201–219. https://doi.org/10.1007/s11256-005-0009-z

Beyond the Black, Brown, and White: Locating Self in Third Spaces in Social Justice Education

Lana Kim and Wonyoung Cho

In the United States (U.S.), race is a core organizing construct that impacts our identities, ways of being, experiences, and relationships. As family therapy clinicians, educators, and scholars with an Asian phenotype, we undoubtedly experience the salience of race play out in cross-racial dynamics with clients, colleagues, administrators, and students. Yet conversations about cross-racial relationships tend to center around the racial binary, highlighting racial tensions as existing between Black/Brown (more recently referred to as Black, Indigenous, and People of Color; BIPOC) and white communities.

However, this obscures the complex ways in which "racial stains and strains" (Hardy, 2008, p. 81) also play out within cross-racial relationships among communities of color. Hardy's (2008) metaphor of "racial stains'' refers to the way in which racially charged events in history inevitably shape the context in which cross-racial relationships are subsequently formed and negotiated in the present. Thereby, "racial stains'' often undergird "racial strains" that get enacted through "polite, cautious, conflict- and intimacy-avoidant, non-trusting but semi-functional interactions that take place among members of diverse racial groups" (p. 81). It speaks to fragility in relationships and points to the need for acknowledging and working through contextual stains in order to create opportunities for meaningful and authentic cross-racial interactions.

As one and a half and second-generation cis-gender women of East Asian descent, race has been an undeniable direct entry point of our engagement into social justice work and one through which both our personal and professional lives intersect. However, our racialized Asian-American identity as well as our unique sociocultural identity are invisibilized or omitted from the dominant racial discourse

L. Kim (✉) · W. Cho
Lewis & Clark College, Portland, OR, USA
e-mail: lkim@lclark.edu; wonyoungcho@lclark.edu

© American Family Therapy Academy (AFTA) 2023

L. A. Nice, C. Eppler (eds.), *Social Justice and Systemic Family Therapy Training*,
AFTA SpringerBriefs in Family Therapy, https://doi.org/10.1007/978-3-031-29930-8_3

of the U.S. where the Black/Brown versus white binary prevails. Therefore, we operate from a structural position referred to as Third Space. In this chapter, we will explore the sociocultural and sociopolitical context of Asian-American realities and discuss how we engage in cross-racial work from Third Space.

1 Socioculturally Locating Asian-Americans in the U.S. Racial Discourse

Identity and belonging are complex topics for Asian-Americans, in part because of the racialized lens through which they are seen societally. This tendency to "other" Asian-Americans is attributable to long-standing representation in media and text that paints persons with Asian phenotypes as forever foreigners or honorary whites, regardless of migration status or birthplace (Tuan, 1998). This dominant narrative is deeply rooted in the sociopolitical history of the U.S., as seen through the Chinese Exclusion Act of 1882, the internment of Japanese Americans in 1942, discriminatory, pre-1965 immigration policies that placed head taxes and quotas on immigrants from Asian countries (Lee, 2015), the Asian-American Movement following the Civil Rights Movement in the 1970s and the 1980s (Takaki, 1998) and again in the early 2000s when South Asian communities were targeted for their phenotypical similarities to the identified terrorists of the September 11, 2001, attacks.

The COVID-19 pandemic and global health crisis in the spring of 2020 speculated to be associated with activities in Wuhan, China, became a catalyst to reignite dormant, racist Yellow Peril (Kawai, 2005) anti-Asian sentiment in the U.S. This coincided with the unjust killing of George Floyd, triggering an increase in the nation's racial consciousness in the midst of escalating political tensions around the national strategy to mitigate the pandemic spread. The resulting racial justice uprising that took hold included attention to the exponential increase in Asian-American and Pacific Islander (AAPI) hate crimes. Thus, the racial discourse in the U.S. started to actually include the nuanced AAPI experience.

Emergent sociological phenomena like this new attention to AAPI issues broadens the binary Black/Brown versus white dominant racial discourse. However, the historical tendency to lump Asian-Americans into the general category of BIPOC relates to the systemic effects of white supremacy: when whiteness is centered in systems, the illusion of BIPOC solidarity prevails. This misses the on-going complexities that have to be negotiated in cross-racial interactions. We see this occur at all societal levels including institutions of higher education.

During my first year as a tenure-track faculty at a Predominantly White Institution (PWI) in the Pacific Northwest of the U.S., I (WC) saw a flier for an affinity group for students of color with the slogan "is it hard being a Black and Brown face in a white place?" Though this question was meant to foster inclusivity and connection for members of the BIPOC community, it inadvertently invisibilized and excluded the experience and identity of Asian-American persons like me. This assumption of the racial binary implies that I as an East Asian-American am invisible, which aligns with the strand of racial discrimination that Asian-Americans often face in the U.S. (Kao, 2006). These seemingly small cross-racial microaggressions often go unacknowledged, which contributes further strain to racial stains (Hardy, 2008).

2   Finding Third Space

Knowledge is culturally and historically specific (Burr, 2015). This applies to racial discourse and the way it shapes our personal and professional lives given our social, cultural, and historical locations. Our geographical contexts, the sociopolitical events we have lived through, our sociocultural conditioning, and our personal and familial immigration history shape our distinct experience of race. As Asian-Americans, we (LK and WC) share many phenotypic identity markers as well as our ethnic (Korean) heritage. However, our contextual realities are distinct and these differences have impacted our respective worldviews and experiences.

Third Space is a term from bilingual education that describes a hybrid learning space where multiple languages, knowledges, and sociocultural scripts are "mutually appropriated" for a more expansive and creative learning outside of a binary framework (Gutiérrez, 2008, p. 153). We use this construct as a conceptual framework to understand our cultural and racial identity; as East Asian-Americans, we do not have a place in the racial binary that dominates U.S. racial conversations. Being persons outside of this binary, we have had to negotiate our own Third Space in these dialogues.

I (LK) am a Canadian-born, cisgender, Asian woman who moved to the U.S. in my adulthood and, consequently, I often feel like a visitor in this country. Even after having lived in the U.S. for over 15 years, the visceral feeling of being an outsider remains. My formative experiences of race and cross-racial relations took place in the context of contemporary 1980s/1990s Vancouver, British Columbia, during a robust time of immigration for many ethnic and racial groups. The embodied experiences of cross-race relationships I have had as an Asian-Canadian woman in Vancouver include explicitly observed racism toward indigenous communities, discrimination against South and East Asian communities, and cross-racial violence; but also neighborly comradery between prominent ethnic minority groups. This set of experiences serve as a noticeably different reference point to my lived and studied learnings about cross-racial relations in the U.S. I experience racism as real, but with the understanding that it is a much more multicultural and nuanced phenomenon than what the U.S. portrays to be a Black/Brown versus white binary issue.

Given this, it has been a challenge to locate myself in the U.S. racial dialogue. I feel both othered as well as conditionally included in the BIPOC discourse. Therefore, I am constantly exploring the boundaries around where I fit versus where and how I need to stand in allyship to other communities of color. It has been critical for me to deepen my historical understanding of racism in this country to navigate my own privilege and marginalization and the accompanying stains and strains that exist with racialized others. For me, occupying Third Space happens through straddling many identities as a bicultural person.

Similarly, my (WC) experiences in engaging with racial dialogues accentuates my outsider status to this country's narrative. This is not an inaccurate representation; I am a one and a half generation immigrant, which means that I was born and socialized in my early childhood in another country and immigrated into the U.S. while I was still young enough to be socialized by the culture of my new home. Since moving to the U.S. in the early 1990s, I continue to be asked by various audiences in my personal and professional life to share my Korean culture and speak on behalf of my people. I understand these invitations to be well-intentioned, yet it is both inviting and alienating: I am reminded of and celebrated for where I come from, while simultaneously remaining a foreigner. This sentiment remains now, decades later, even though I have lived longer in the U.S. than any other country in the world.

Very early on in my life, I came to accept and embrace my non-belongingness. I was too Korean for the Asian-Americans, too American for the Koreans, and definitely not American enough for the Americans. The non-belonging to any of these racialized identities may have started from subtle rejections, but I coped by making it an intentional and personal stance. I spent significant portions of my life maintaining my Korean language, learning Korean history, and consuming Korean media such as K-pop, talk shows, dramas, and movies; in other words, intentionally defining my non-belongingness. This was possible in part due to the time in which I grew up. With the rise of the personal computer in the mid to late 1990s and early 2000s, the Internet provided instantaneous global connection. Soon, I found myself in a new learning space, a "Third Space," that connected me to contemporary cultural information of both Korea and the U.S. There I was able to find my audience and community with whom I felt a sense of belonging – a community of transnationals, internationals, and others who did not quite fit in the sociocultural context of their geographical location. Thus, even from thousands of miles away, I was able to keep up relatively well with Korean culture and its evolving language in real time. I was, and am, intentionally and biculturally transnational.

3   Learning to Teach from Third Space

As authors who are explicitly examining the construct of race as it relates to our training and experiences with teaching and clinical work, we are aware that our respective birth places of South Korea (WC) and Canada (LK) and subsequent immigration contexts and timeframes acutely shape our experiences of existing as Asian-Americans in Third Spaces. We also reflect on our formal family therapy education and training in the mid- to late-2000s and notice that we came up in the field during a generation where postmodernism and social constructionism (Gergen, 1999) were privileged and conversations about race were just starting to get broached. As such, social justice terminology and concepts related to racial diversity were in development as were the ideas about how to engage in these discussions. Our graduate experiences around conversations about race centered around the Black/Brown and white binary or ones where we felt lumped into the category of BIPOC and thus expected to generally speak to it. So, how have these experiences influenced our work around race as Asian-American marriage and family therapy educators learning to teach from Third Space?

My (LK) learning related to engaging in conversations around race and cross-racial differences from Third Space has been experientially driven. For me, these lessons have always occurred spontaneously within the relational context with students. As I continue to navigate and facilitate conversations about race, I am taken back to a formative early experience in my teaching career when I was instructing a course focused specifically on the integration of diversity, equity, and inclusion (DEI) in family therapy. At the time, I was a core faculty member teaching in the southeast region of the U.S. among a tight-knit team of colleagues who held intersections of diversity in their social locations and aligned with diversity, equity, and inclusion aims, but who did so from their embodied identities as white people. Thus, in our program with racially diverse students, approximately 50% who identified as white and 50% students of color who predominantly identified as Black or African American, I represented the sole, ethnically diverse faculty presence.

Because of the racial diversity among the student body, when it came to discussing the topic of race and racism, students were able to share from both a personal and theoretical space. However, I quickly learned that in order to create a context for this to happen, I had to lead with carefully planned pedagogical exercises to foster connection. I also needed to intentionally model risk taking and holding tension for different realities. One particular week I decided to assign students to asynchronously watch Lee's (1994) documentary film, *The Color of Fear*, before attending class. This was an assignment that previous instructors of the course had assigned to other cohorts which provided stimulating content for class discussion on race. The 1994 documentary film features eight cisgender men of European, Latino, Asian, and African descent who passionately engage in personal discussions about race relations in the U.S. The class objective that week was to debrief students' thoughts and reflections about the film, examine connections to their own lives, and apply the content to the clinical context.

The in-class conversation started similarly to how it might typically be expected – generalized observations about racism and cross-racial tension that still exist in current day, some statements denouncing racism from white students who were trying to navigate their privileged positionality, white fragility, and demonstrated allyship, and some personal examples from students of color about the relevance of the film's content to their present day lives and society at large. While there was friction around the film's content and topic, I felt cautiously optimistic about the potential for the dialogue process to deepen. At the same time, I noticed the closed-off body posture and demonstrable silence shown by one of the most vocal students in the class, who was also a Black man. Any attempts I made to specifically engage this student's voice were ignored and met with increasing tension.

I was thrown off by this because of the strong rapport I thought this student and I had shared, which contrasted from the rejecting stance he was taking. The student's dismissiveness toward me and the general tension he demonstrated in the conversation was also felt by the other students who kept glancing in his direction throughout the class period. Eventually, I took a risk and publicly acknowledged his silence stating that it seemed meaningful and that I was interested to know what he was thinking and feeling. He took a lingering pause and then stood up and passionately began explaining the pain and rage the film had brought up for him and the irritation and anger he felt toward me for facilitating the conversation in a way that assumed a level of safety that in fact did not exist for him. He proceeded to name the cross-racial stains that existed between Black/African American communities like his and Asian communities like mine. He cited socio-historical events such as the 1992 Rodney King murder and subsequent Los Angeles riots that had left significant stains on the cross-racial dynamics between Black and Asian communities. Finally, he shared personally about the covert and overt racist experiences he had endured throughout his life by Asian identified women who suspiciously tracked him in their stores or restaurants or the way they clutched their purses and tried to avoid walking near him on the streets.

I felt embarrassed, angry, and apologetic for how he had been treated by members of my race. Additionally, a part of me also felt defensive about the discriminatory experiences he was projecting onto me. But ultimately, I appreciated the lesson he was helping me learn about what needs to be brought into conversations about race in order to expand the dominant discourse around the Black and Brown versus white racial binary. This interaction also helped me recognize the effects of the socialization I had received around cross-racial dynamics as a person who operated from Third Space. I realized that as a second-generation Korean-Canadian coming from outside U.S. culture, and seen as such, I tended to enter into cross-racial interactions with an assumption of shared understanding to persons I perceived to also hold marginalized identities when that connection had not been established. I perpetuated the racial binary by assuming that people of color were allies at face value. I had not addressed the racial stains and strains in the cross-racial context surrounding this student and me and took for granted that students like him would feel a sense of safety and trust with instructors like me just by virtue of our shared BIPOC status.

This experience taught me that conversations about race need to be directly contextualized to the persons in it and that the backdrop of experiences we have in relation to one another exist as stains to be discussed. In retrospect, I should have acknowledged that in the U.S., racial discourse often excludes or overlooks the cross-racial tensions that can lie beneath the surface of presumed BIPOC allyship. I would also have discussed how our experience talking about race is not only shaped by the larger context of systemic racism, but also our own histories of cross-racial interactions and relationships as well as the direct and indirect experiences we have had of racism given our unique contexts. Subsequently, I would have described how my upbringing and experiences in Canada as a second generation Korean-Canadian person with a multicultural social network had informed the reactions that came up for me while watching *The Color of Fear* and the reflections I was bringing into the class conversation. I would have shared that I held an underlying assumption that BIPOC individuals would feel safer to discuss race with other BIPOC individuals, and that I needed to be cognizant of how this false assumption could mislead my facilitation of the conversation. I could have highlighted that while there is a need to explicitly address cross-racial nuances in conversations about racism, we struggle in part because this is often left out and there is no template for how to engage with it. Cross-racial dynamics need to be intentionally broached in conversations about race and race relations to move toward inclusivity and change.

I (WC) "debuted" officially as faculty in the fall semester of 2019 at a Marriage, Couple, and Family Therapy (MCFT) program as the waves of the recent rapid sociocultural and political shifts began. My experiences as a clinical supervisor and adjunct instructor prior to this time provided me with a solid footing of pedagogy and teaching practices, but the onslaught of sociopolitical changes sparked by the global Covid-19 pandemic and the racial justice movements reignited by the tragic murder of George Floyd quickly and dramatically shifted my role as an educator. This role shift was not intentional or internally motivated, and I felt the changes with how students seemed to relate to me as their instructor even before I settled into my first full-time faculty appointment. A significant portion of my challenge as an Asian-American female instructor prior to these changes was to fight the invisibility and be seen, and to prove myself as a knowledgeable and trustworthy authority and evaluator. However, the ground under my feet quickly shifted; I felt hyper-visible as a woman of color (as in not-white) and found myself managing students' desperate and anxious desire to garner my approval.

There were many complicating factors influencing this: navigating the new world of online learning with all of its general uncertainty and conflicting information, a dramatic increase of socioemotional impacts due to physical isolation and "shelter in place" protocols, and the general unrest resulting from breakdown of daily life and an uncertain future. This, in conjunction with the rapid and intense attention to racial justice issues rumbling underneath the American social consciousness, the students, especially those who are or can pass as white, seemed eager to prove to me that they were not "one of those white people" – those who commit racial and social injustice.

In the foundational family therapy theories course, students are evaluated on their mastery of chosen theories through a case conceptualization paper based on a family or relational unit from a movie. I ask students to offer a movie they would like to use for this assignment each year, and the class collectively chooses one from those their peers have suggested. Recently, students have started to volunteer Korean (foreign) and Korean-American made (domestic) movies. Each of these years, at least one class chose the distinctly Korean movies – *Parasite* (Bong, 2019) in 2020 and *Minari* (Chung, 2021) in 2021. Perhaps this is partially due to the increase in accessibility and popularity of South Korean media in recent years, however it strikes me as more than coincidental that students offer and select these films to write their paper with me, and that they intentionally select these because of my Korean-American identity.

Once the students start applying theory and attempt to socioculturally attune to the families in these movies, they inevitably start to ask questions and I find myself in the familiar position of being asked to explain on behalf of my people, who are sometimes Korean, sometimes Korean-American, and sometimes Asian-American. The students start to experience the daunting task of having to learn enough about Korean culture within an academic semester to demonstrate competence in socioculturally attuning their theories and interventions. They start feeling the pressure to prove to me, their evaluator and a perceived insider of these cultures, that they did enough to legitimize themselves as culturally competent. Moreover, they express anxiety in not wanting to offend me as the evaluator but also the insider and a representative of the culture they are attempting to attune to.

I have started to clarify what the students' learning objectives are in these moments, namely, that they are not to learn Korean culture. Rather, the learning objectives are to hold the not-knowing stance that is needed when working with racially and culturally diverse clientele while bearing the tension of wanting to do right by them but knowing that we can never fully know. They are to creatively brainstorm how to move forward competently, ethically, and continuously attuning. Here, I teach from the Third Space both personally and professionally: personally, in that I show up as not quite Korean and not quite American, and facilitate conversations with the students about the complexity of the hyphenated experience of being Asian-American; professionally in that therapists will never quite fully know where their clients come from. I have found that, so far, this Third Space allows me to provide a bit of grace as the white-adjacent to the white students who are anxious to do right by the BIPOC, to empathize with the Black and Brown students as an honorary BIPOC, and to validate those students who do not fit in the racial binary. Inviting the students into this Third Space with me has been instrumental in encouraging them to think about race more expansively, and thus more inclusively.

4 Application to Teaching and Practice

As East Asian-American educators teaching from Third Space, there are several practical applications that we take from our experiences into teaching and clinical contexts. First, it is necessary to help students understand and differentiate both the larger social context of racism as well as the unique ways in which one's racial experiences are socioculturally and locally specific. Zooming in and out from Third Space location can bring forth unique vantage points as well as help counter invisibility and highlight unseen biases in the self-of-the-therapist learning process. It also introduces greater nuance to conversations about race which steers participants away from reifying a static discourse around power and privilege. When instructors who operate from Third Space engage in this practice, they can help students engage with self and others in more meaningful and transformative ways.

For us, a major part of teaching and practicing from Third Space centers around our identity as East Asian-Americans who exist outside of the Black/Brown and white binary. Part of how we bring our identity forward from Third Space is by resisting the seduction of co-opting the Black/Brown struggle and instead define and speak truth to our own unique experiences as East Asian-Americans in a racially dichotomous society. This requires intentional focus around self-of-the-educator development relative to one's racial history through time, place, and sociocultural context. To this end, we encourage the following points of reflection to facilitate this self-of-the-educator growing edge.

First, we believe it is important to learn about the racial history of East Asian-Americans in the U.S. as well as disentangle it from the larger Asian diaspora. For example, it is important to understand how U.S. immigration policies have created immigration trends for Asian-Americans at large and the attitudes of the American public toward these groups. These experiences are diverse within the Asian-American community as their involuntary/voluntary migration pathways are impacted heavily by social class, education level, and colorism. These attitudes subsequently influence the systemic oppression that our ethnic communities have differentially experienced.

Second, contextualize one's unique family history and journey of immigration within the global and U.S. landscape. For example, families immigrating to the U.S. in the late 1960s and 1970s have vastly different cultural and sociopolitical stories than the families immigrating in the 1990s and early 2000s. The implications of the time and space of entry to the U.S. greatly shapes our positionalities and experiences of power and privilege as members of society.

Third, recognize ways in which one's positionality as an East Asian-American today intersects with the larger BIPOC experience, while acknowledging how the relative levels of privilege and oppression differ in relation to race. It is also important to know and acknowledge nodal events that have shaped cross-racial relations in the U.S.

We anticipate that the evolving racial dialogue in the U.S. will continue to broaden and include focus on intra- and cross-racial dynamics involving various ethnicities and multiethnic identities. This paradigm shift is in motion and educators can fuel the momentum by diversifying the way we facilitate racial justice conversations. One way to do this is by introducing social constructs such as Third Space in conversations about race and identity. Rather than over-identifying with simplified, static, and totalizing racial narratives, racial justice conversations should facilitate deeper examination of how these complex intersections of sociocultural, political, and historical narratives intersect in the lives of the individuals participating in these conversations. Another way is to include content in the curriculum that engages students to reflect upon and examine the ways in which unacknowledged cross-racial stains and strains present in their own lives and communities and the macro sociocultural context. Engaging in conversations such as these can center the non-white experience, introduce nuance to the BIPOC experience, and offer new ground for transformative societal processes to take place from Third Space.

Furthermore, in cross-racial dialogue, showing up authentically requires a willingness to directly bring educator-as-self into the conversation and utilize the dynamics that are created with students in live time given the interplay between the educator and students' identities. As educators, we need to model what it looks like to courageously and compassionately broach direct dialogue around sociocultural, and perhaps more personal, stains and strains that exist cross-racially. We need to model what it means to acknowledge aspects of our identity that connect to others' privilege as well as their marginalization. We posit that the way toward racial justice comes from honest and personal reckoning with the racial stains and strains, and from deep collective wrestling with the complex reality of how the racial discourses of the U.S. touch each of us. We view this work as continuous and evolving.

References

Burr, V. (2015). *Social constructionism* (3rd ed.). Routledge. https://doi.org/10.4324/9781315715421

Gergen, K. J. (1999). *An invitation to social construction* (1st ed.). Sage.

Gutiérrez, K. D. (2008). Developing a Sociocritical literacy in the third space. *Reading Research Quarterly, 43*(2), 148–164. https://doi.org/10.1598/RRQ.43.2.3

Hardy, K. (2008). Race, reality, and relationships: Implications for the re-visioning of family therapy. In M. McGoldrick & K. Hardy (Eds.), *Re-visioning family therapy: Race, culture, and gender in clinical practice* (2nd ed., pp. 76–84). The Guilford Press.

Kao, G. (2006). Where are the Asian and Hispanic victims of Katrina? A metaphor for invisible minorities in contemporary racial discourse. *Du Bois Review: Social Science Research on Race, 3*(1), 223–231. https://doi.org/10.1017/S1742058X06060152

Kawai, Y. (2005). Stereotyping Asian Americans: The dialectic of the model minority and the yellow peril. *The Howard Journal of Communication, 16*, 109–130. https://doi.org/10.1080/10646170590948974

Lee, M. (2015). *The making of Asian America: A history.* Simon & Schuster.

Takaki, R. (1998). *A history of Asian Americans: Strangers from a different shore.* Bay Back Books.

Tuan, M. (1998). *Forever foreigners or honorary whites? The Asian ethnic experience today.* Rutgers University Press.

Relational Social Justice: Looking in the Mirror with Others Bearing Witness

Matthew R. Mock

For many of us, working in the community began as, and continues to be, a contribution to social justice. My decades of work for social justice as a practitioner and educator of therapists, educators, and other healers have afforded me many gifts. One of these is insights to ways we can engage across differences to connect us with others for greater equity and fairness. Providing therapeutic services and training others for sensitive, welcomed work within communities will be my legacy. Working through public mental health settings means working with people most in need who have the least resources. During the ongoing health pandemic, inequities and unfairness have become more pronounced and even exacerbated. Housing, health care, food and nutrition, employment, education, social services, and foundational civil rights are not automatic "givens." What many of us thought to be civil rights finally won are the focus of battles to be fought once more.

Many families, with whom we work so hard to forge therapeutic alliances and working relationships, are oftentimes poor or underemployed, or at the precipice of some life circumstance. Many have faced multiple losses or traumas or are multi-oppressed, experiencing little in the way of influence or real, sustained power. Mutual trust and respect are highly valued. Many Black, Indigenous, People of Color (BIPOC) will encounter racial traumas throughout our lifetimes. We have figuratively had to hold our breath for the next act of racism or bias to be experienced, directly or indirectly. As we have witnessed, some individuals have had their breathing restricted by unequally treating systems such as law enforcement, education, health services, and employment. Some, such as George Floyd and Breonna Taylor, died at the hands of individuals supposedly representing justice systems.

M. R. Mock (✉)
JFK School of Psychology of National University, Pleasant Hill, CA, USA
e-mail: mmock@nu.edu

© American Family Therapy Academy (AFTA) 2023
L. A. Nice, C. Eppler (eds.), *Social Justice and Systemic Family Therapy Training*,
AFTA SpringerBriefs in Family Therapy, https://doi.org/10.1007/978-3-031-29930-8_4

Clearly, victims of systemic inequities have been held down from opportunities in life. Having our breathing restricted is akin to constricting our human spirit.

I view my work as an educator in the community as one of the primary ways in which I confront injustice and create space for the human spirit to grow. In this chapter, I will describe some of the particular life experiences that have especially impacted my journey into this work, my approach to first "looking in the mirror" and sharing these reflections with students, and finally different ways that I "invite others to witness" as I support them in their own growth. My own growth is also never ending.

1   Acknowledgement of Our Self, Family, and Social Location

I find it essential to be aware of the foundations of our own cultural selves as we do the work of social justice and advocacy. We benefit from recognizing our own social location and ways our lives have been shaped in early development. I identify myself as a third generation, Chinese-American, heterosexual, able-bodied, cisgender male. I grew up in a large family (the middle child of seven children across a 14-year age span) and was raised lower working class. Having enough food for each meal was sometimes a challenge. My hard-working Chinese-American father served the community as a highly dedicated postal worker. My fairly mono-lingual, Cantonese-dialect speaking mother worked raising us in our small home, doing her best to make those limited meals. While one might say my family was economically stretched or poor, we were intensely immersed in valued relationships of family and siblings. In this way, I felt relationally enriched. My interactions with my siblings also created questions that I would pursue as I grew older. Why were my two sisters treated differently than the boys? Why were jokes told about some ethnic groups considered funny, while jabs taken at my own Asian-American identity were hurtful? Learning was multifaceted. For as long as I could recall, education was always highly valued as a means to better one's future and the reputation of my family. I was one of the first in my family to complete an undergraduate degree. I am the only one to earn master and doctoral degrees. No matter what, throughout my life I have always been reminded about humility while growing up in my home.

I have been highly influenced by several sources throughout my life. Some of these major influences include strong Asian women, civil rights leaders, and ordinary people with extraordinary things to convey. These were often racial or ethnic individuals, young and old, with some who were willing to sacrifice their lives to share their truths. Growing up in a largely white community in West Los Angeles, I longed to hear from people who were more like me; people of color. The civil rights and peace movements framed my social and educational experience. As with so many children, by default the television acted as a babysitter of sorts. Witnessing injustices, political unrest and violence related to war, and protest movements for peace and equity were undeniable realities on the nightly news. My older brothers were enamored with folk, rock, and soul music of the time. Television and music on the radio served as cultural windows and mirrors. Social justice and the fights for equity were not just for me to see but also to hear; to experience viscerally.

Our family was one of the few in my community and early schooling who were of Chinese descent. My first significant partner was a Jewish woman. I was 15 years old. We learned about what it meant to be in an inter-racial relationship, still uncommon at that time. It was from her that I learned about the Holocaust, the importance of root or home culture, and not forgetting ancestral histories. The 1960s and 1970s were significant periods of racial unrest and social protests long overdue. Activism for social justice was at a high, not just as talk, but actual action to consider. Witnessing and taking part in such protests, painful as well as triumphant, would leave me with an indelible impression. Those who I was drawn to, and those drawn to me for support, shared similar passions and willingness to question authority.

2 The Foundation of Our Work: Social Justice as a Process of "Looking in the Mirror" at Oneself and Others

In a naïve way, cultural competence was often thought of and even portrayed as learning about cultural others (i.e., working "outside-in"). In its worst form, this might be seen as some form of voyeurism or anthropological appropriation. Even at its best, cultural competence means understanding a client's cultural background and influences from an outsider's perspective. While this approach might support a good working relationship, it may also pose a "working for" rather than "working with" mentality. Cultural humility, on the other hand for me, poses a stance of "not knowing," of holding oneself accountable, and, in some ways, "looking into the mirror" at oneself. Social injustices are often not just unique one-time situations; rather they are ones that occur as part of a pattern of repeated mistreatment of micro- or macro-aggressions against others. With injustices replicated and sustained in systems it must be asked in what ways as individuals are we victims, witnesses, or perpetrators of such inequities? In this way, I think of a process of teaching about social justice as needing to look at oneself in the mirror with others bearing witness. Looking in the mirror means being aware of one's own identity and social location, power, and privilege, and impact through societal 'isms. It also means having others bear witness to what we are seeing and experiencing, and being accountable to our perceptions.

3 Use of "Self" in the Process of Teaching for Social Justice

Strategically sharing one's own life experiences can be beneficial for educating others. I often share with students that I grew up during the era of social protests and civil rights. Seeing African Americans being chased, hosed down or struck with batons, or worse, by riot police had a profound impact on me. Seeing and listening to the passionate pleas of Martin Luther King, Jr., and Malcolm X left indelible impressions that I would take into my later career and life. Longing for peace during the Vietnam War, icons like Gandhi, Mother Teresa, and protestor Daniel Ellsberg formed ideas that I would follow. As a young adult, I was disturbed by the racially motivated killing of Vincent Chin, a Chinese-American man on the eve of his wedding in Michigan. Mistaken as Japanese by unemployed auto workers in Detroit, he was stalked and killed. When the presiding judge allowed the perpetrators to go free with no jail time and only a paltry monetary fine, I was outraged. Ironically, my eventual career came about as a result of protests as well as resistance.

The generation I grew up in influenced my view of social justice. As a senior at Brown University, I worked in a study lab with a young psychology professor. Because he was also new to teaching and learning, he was open to exploring questions together. My assignment was shadowing one of two autistic twin boys, observing and charting their behaviors. At the time, aversive conditioning was being utilized. For instance, when there were undesirable behaviors being shown such as mild head banging or self-biting, the young boy was given mild electric shock. I recall being repulsed by what I thought was unjust and unethical treatment. My professor welcomed my reactions. It was then that I decided to go into the field of psychology and psychotherapy to contribute to more just and humane interventions. This professor who guided my thinking and sensitivity is a member of my professional genogram. Subsequently, even more significant are individuals who quickly shaped my career practicing therapy. There were strong, feminist Asian scholars and highly respected practitioners such as Evelyn Lee, Reiko True, Christine Iijima-Hall, and later, Jean Lau Chin. Robert Jay Green, founder of the Rockway Institute for Lesbian, Gay, Bisexual, Transgender (LGBT) Psychology, recommended me to the American Family Therapy Academy (AFTA), not only as a new member but as one to receive the annual social justice and diversity award. This was early in my career. It was also at AFTA meetings that I met Monica McGoldrick and Nydia Garcia Preto, who were life changing for me, furthering my passions. They were to become my professional, chosen family members. Sharon C Ngim, an attorney and my wife, concretized mutual commitments for "serving community needs" at all levels.

Through my professional family, not only was I asked to share my thinking on treatment of diverse families, I was also invited to write book chapters and present at annual conferences at the Multicultural Family Institute of New Jersey (MFINJ). Being welcomed into a professional family deeply committed to diversity and social justice with an ability to not only teach embedded principles within them, but also discuss them, was and remains invaluable to this very day. For my own biological family of Chinese heritage and ancestry, injustices were witnessed and often to be endured in order to "pass" or be accepted as new immigrants. With this additional new family and community I could be myself, question unfairness, test out ideas, share my outrage, and protest against acts of racism, sexism, classism, inequities, and more. My passionate ideas about fairness, equity, and justice were allowed a place to be shared with similar others. I "found my voice" and was able to finally open up, let go to be my genuine self, even to celebrate when I was understood. I found connection and community. In turn, I want to pass this experience on to others.

4 Creating a Context for Learning and Relational Engagement

I hold a perspective that social justice is a lifelong commitment with teaching embodying a deeply meaningful context for learning. I have found it essential to establish and maintain an environment for safe, relational, socially just education among students by creating "learning agreements." These agreements commonly include confidentiality, speaking from an "I" place with self and other accountability, being aware of occupied space during shared interactions, maintaining full presence, listening and talking with mutual respect, agreeing to disagree, engaging in dialogue rather than debate, using mindfulness for self and others, and striving to embody personal and professional compassion. Astute skills in group process for modeling these learning agreements, reiterating them and pointing them out strategically goes a long way in establishing safety and trust for rich, authentic interactions. The interchanges that follow are often deeply meaningful and memorable.

I have previously written extensively, and in detail, about powerful ways for teaching diversity and social justice (Mock, 2019). In that chapter I describe the overview I use to effectively train students on related principles of diversity and cultural competence, as well as humility, social location, intersectionality, and social justice. I also speak of preparing for situations of anticipated challenge. These are critical opportunities for new educational experiences. Learning agreements – framing and consistently embodying and demonstrating them – are essential. Again, these agreements frame critical stances and an enduring environment to share experiences.

5 Calling Others "Out" to Bring Them "In" for Critical Learning

Racial and cultural communities have experiences related to social justice on a daily basis. These experiences can be dynamically brought into teaching spaces and places. As an example of ways such courses can be so critical to education, I have taught a graduate course titled: "Asian Americans: Socio-cultural and Psychological Perspectives." This course, which I have taught for decades, fulfills a requirement for all doctoral psychology students to take a course centered on one cultural community. I have a range of students, some with personal experiences to differing degrees as Asian Americans, and others who have little or seemingly insignificant experiences as they do not identify as being of Asian ancestry. I often begin with a process of personal centering with learning agreements and sharing of strategic self-narrative.

I teach and have students explore histories related to specific Asian American Pacific Islander Native Hawaiian communities. We even challenge the construction of these politically and socially constructed identities. Questions such as "how are we the same, yet different under such an umbrella?" create rich dialogues. For example, students learn that while being listed under such a heading, Pacific Islanders do not feel fully seen or valued, with some having more experiences reso-nating with those who are Indigenous or Native American. After framing important history as might be done via Asian American or ethnic studies, I then strategically arrange for my students to learn in the field. Berkeley is the original land of the Ohlone. Early learning includes going to Angel Island, which was the home of the Miwok. Angel Island was also the first checkpoint for laborers from China, not only seeking work but a new home. The Chinese Exclusion Act of 1882 was the first race-based legislation unjustly focusing on one cultural group for immigration. I also facilitate my students "learning deeply in context" in Japantown, where the majority of Japanese-American residents in the early 1940s lined up to report to internment camps under Executive Order 9066. Students may study ayurvedic med-icine via a South Asian practitioner or have a meal in the Little Saigon Vietnamese community in San Francisco speaking with an elder or young person about their identity and life or family experiences. Inevitably historical and racial trauma arise in such stories of immigration or being a refugee, or of mistreatment and social injustices via racism and other negative social forces of marginalization and not being fully valued.

For some, these immersion experiences may evoke feelings of guilt, shame, or being "intruders" or even "voyeurs." Facilitating and sharing dialogues about this are often valuable. Timely discussions about the history of colonization and how it has been and is manifested are key. Addressing white guilt and fragility are also necessary to confront inequities. This is where reminders of cultural humility and empathy, even taking them to radical levels as through the work of liberation psy-chology (Comas-Díaz & Torres Rivera, 2020), are very significant.

No matter where I go, there is no absence of teaching about history and diversity, and therefore lessons centered on social justice. It is more a matter of "to what degree." Making dormant perspectives come alive or raising new consciousness impacts learners in lasting ways that they retain for their subsequent work. No mat-ter what and where, I reference lessons cutting across communities. How does prior Chinese exclusion relate to current anti-immigrant rhetoric? How were African-American and Japanese-American communities brought together during the intern-ment camps? How were Indigenous, Native American communities viewed as less than human or used as scapegoats as were early Asian immigrants? How did the Bracero Program bring in laborers from Mexico but only temporarily to fill a labor void? When Japanese-American farm workers were interned during World War II, workers from other countries including Mexico were brought in to pick the crops. But these workers were not allowed to stay as immigrants. How does this relate to current debates and struggles regarding undocumented workers versus those welcomed into the United States with open arms as new immigrants? I, as well as students, have found the many discussions and interchanges that follow such questions to be deeply meaningful as well as memorable.

6   Use of Self to Assist Others to Look More Deeply

At particular junctures of our mutual learning experience, I often model storytelling for my participants. It is my belief that, if we cannot perform things we ask of others, change is more difficult and less authentic. Knowing the "self-of-the-therapist" is essential. I selectively share some of my own stories as a Chinese-American growing up in a predominantly white, middle-class community in Los Angeles. My fellow learners inevitably become more engaged, often feeling safer to tell their own stories using the learning agreements I have established. Sometimes, at a particular juncture toward the end of the class, I work with the class by sharing a story of a social situation that appeared to be an incident of discrimination. I share the story of an Asian-American man similar to myself who seemed to be mistreated in a department store. As he tried to make a purchase in the store, he was regarded by the white salesperson as though he were not there. When she did attend to him, she interacted with him with suspicion as a "foreigner" who was out of place, not to be trusted. After he protested, she put the problem back on him, demeaning him by speaking slowly, as though English were not his first language (although it was) and insisting he not cause trouble. I ask attendees to consider why they might decide whether this was an act of discrimination (i.e., due to race, class, communication differences) or not, giving potential alternative explanations (such as, the man had been rude previous to the incident, a warning had been out that a man fitting his description had been a problem earlier; etc.). Together we try to construct the potential story and deconstruct it in order to consider how we might have intervened. In the end, I eventually reveal that I was that Asian-American man who was treated unfairly with discrimination.

The majority of participants often react with surprise, dismay, or even shock. Most come away from the story with greater understanding of how pervasive and insidious mistreatment through social inequities and power differentials can be even among those they may assume to be immune. As a highly regarded, highly acculturated, and educated professor they expect me to be treated with respect. But due to racism and stereotypes, I am not always treated as such. Rather than being culturally competent, the students experience and often react in ways appreciating cultural humility and personal compassion. Occasionally crossing paths with a few participants years later, they often tell me how they remember this story and disclosure. In summary, when teachers authentically share some of their own narratives, their teaching or vision for social justice becomes even more vivid and palpable because it is more easily relatable as well as memorable.

While I always have a teaching plan, ripe opportunities arise for powerful learning spontaneously. My class topic for an afternoon was on racial violence, historically and in the current context. As I was preparing for teaching in the morning, the following occurred on a street near the University of California, Berkeley campus: I heard a woman scream "You almost ran me over!" As I got closer to the scene, a middle-aged white man driving a pickup truck was shouting derogatory racial epithets directed toward the woman, who appeared to be a South Asian university student. As she was crossing the street with flashing crossing lights, the man had nearly struck her with his truck while cursing at her. He then stepped out of his truck verbally threatening her. As an ally to the woman, I thought quickly about the "Hollaback" intervention strategies I learned online to disarm racial situations. I first shouted out to bring the situation to the attention of other bystanders. I then quickly assisted the woman to withdraw from the man and his escalating tirade. We quickly went to a safe space close by where there was an officer available to speak with her and ensure her safety. The conversation an hour later about this incident I witnessed was timely; the class discussed the rise of anti-Asian violence during the Covid-19 pandemic, including its origins as well as historical precursors of systemic racism and prejudice.

Teachers must recognize their own held privileges. As an acculturated, heterosexual, able-bodied, middle class, Ivy-league graduate who is a cisgender male, I am seen as having certain advantages. Ways I address issues of gender, sexual orientation, ableism, social and class standing, and immigration might well be instructive to others. Accusations of being "white adjacent" need to be met with a discussion of how white supremacy attempts to divide BIPOC individuals for the benefit of those who have colonized and dominated non-whites. Intra-ethnic differences within groups might need to be addressed as well. I have had several such opportunities.

I recall being asked to speak at the national Asian American and Pacific Islander (AAPI) conference. One of the goals of the conference was to address the diversity and complexity of what it means to be identified under the heading of Asian American and Pacific Islander (AAPI). During my presentation, a woman who identified as indigenous Native Hawaiian did not feel that I, as Chinese American, could speak directly to her cultural identity. This interaction occurred with all conference attendees bearing witness. A subsequent conversation about the background of the AAPI designation with an understanding of the differences among us, including how an umbrella referencing gives strength in numbers in some contexts yet is invisibilizing in others, was very impactful. She shared how she felt more heard and seen, and therefore empowered. We had an open dialogue about this in front of the entire audience. As a result, other conversations took place among attendees. Continuing in my own recent work with AAPIs, I have found it very important to proactively acknowledge our intra-ethnic differences. My personal experience of visiting Guam, for example, has brought to light how colonization has impacted the Chamorros, the indigenous people of the island. While AAPIs may share somewhat in-common experiences, we are certainly not all the same.

7 Common Principles of Teaching Social Justice

Having done this work for decades, it is affirming to remember on an ongoing basis some of the major elements posed for social justice education for therapists in transformative practice. Common principles I always have in mind are to:

1. Balance cognitive, intellectual, factual aspects with emotional connections of the learning process, both shorter and longer term.
2. Acknowledge as well as support the personal experience of participants while bringing to light the systemic interactions among social groups. Concrete real examples brought into consciousness are most often remembered.
3. Attend consistently to social relationships and interactions within the learning situation or classroom. There must be careful observation and noticing of behaviors emerging in group dynamics and exchanges. Rather than blaming or judging conflicts that arise, for example, such interactions should be used for improving interpersonal communications and awareness of processes. These can be powerful moments of learning for future situations.
4. Utilize mindfulness, reflection, and experience for participant-centered learning. Acknowledging one's worldview and experience is often the starting point for problem posing and deep, meaningful ongoing dialogues.
5. Value awareness, personal growth, and change as outcomes of the learning process. Increased personal knowledge, greater social awareness, and making accountable commitments are meaningful stepping-stones to social action. (Bell et al., 2007, pp. 42–43).

8 Making Overarching Commitments and Points of Accountability

Making a commitment as a family therapist or human service provider to social justice in everyday practice is among the hardest work that we do. I am also realistic about the fact that, although the aforementioned trainings can seem transformational in the immediate moment, they may not feel the same in the long term. Attendees often give me feedback that they feel more hopeful, invigorated, and more connected in their commitments to make a difference toward equity in their work with families. While I sincerely commend them for their genuine hard work, I also challenge them about the reality we face; that as we go back to day-to-day life, the social forces that underlie inequities will creep back in and may even undermine their newly constructed commitments to social justice.

As an illustration of this systemic entropy or staying stuck in the same place, I sometimes ask trainees to address a letter to themselves. I have each write a thoughtful, personal note that lists what specific commitments they will make to social justice as family therapists. The commitments must be framed as specific acts, such as "I will point out incidences of sexism as they arise" or "When my family uses derisive language, I will inquire about their meaning" or "When I witness acts that contribute to cycles of mistreatment, I will stand up and interrupt them" or "I will turn political acts of social injustice into opportunities to actively resist and protest in ways that meaningfully involve others." I then take these commitments and put them in self-addressed envelopes. Some months after my teaching session is over, I send these self-written letters back to the trainees. I have had students tell me how powerful their response is on receiving their own letters. They reconsider their own accountability and how hard it is to maintain without consistency. Some will also tell me how liberating it was that they had actually followed through on their commitments.

Social justice work is not to be done alone or in a vacuum. I share this precaution with others while also reminding myself. The demands are high for not just the work itself but all that it entails intellectually, emotionally, relationally, and soulfully. I am often asked what I do as a "soul-healer" to stay healthy, optimistic, vibrant, and forward-thinking in my work. That is another chapter that we as social justice warriors must write, all the more in the context of current, challenging times.

9   Social Justice: Serving Community Needs Personally, Politically, and Professionally

While becoming therapists, we can learn the theories, mechanics, and components of interventions based in theory. Those who teach and practice social justice make connections between knowledge, awareness, and action. I beseech my students to recognize multiple spheres of influence in their daily lives. As they are becoming future family therapists, I challenge them to recognize the power they are taking on and the responsibility they are assuming with every child, adolescent, and family who encounters them. What we actually do with what we learn is the art of therapy. Similarly, the way I use narratives to teach about social justice is not simple or linear; it is a complex art with potentially beautiful results.

While I conduct my work for social justice with humility, affirmations or "booster shots" for our lifelong work, I find "serving community needs" as a welcomed form of ongoing self-care. Noting the positive effects of our work in the community is certainly gratifying. When our community work related to social justice is picked up by others, this can also re-energize us. Serving the community by trying to address their needs can be forever memorable, paving the way for others as well as other opportunities for contributing to greater equity and social justice. In other words, one's own efforts may be found in others who then also carry on the work.

I have this as an example. While attending a community-based conference on race, culture, and practice, a prominent, nationally known, African-American trainer opened by challenging the audience. He pointedly asked how many in the large room felt they were significantly challenged during their graduate training regarding race, especially white therapists, and their holding of power and privilege. Less than a handful raised their hands, and even then, only after a pause. One woman, a white supervisor, stated (my paraphrasing): "I don't know how many people know him, but Dr. Mock was one of my professors where I was trained about community mental health, and I learned a great deal from him." As it turned out, this supervisor did not know that I was sitting in the back of the room. She had been one of my graduate students in required community mental health and multicultural psychology courses. In these courses I share a perspective that working with others is less about us and more about families and communities, and services they need. It had been several years since I had seen this supervisor, and I was truly touched and grateful to know I had such a positive, lasting impact on her. I felt additionally uplifted and inspired to do more. Our work does matter, can multiply among others, and positively contribute to communities.

The work for therapists in furthering social justice has been, is currently, and will be challenging in the future. I remind all that many others came before us and many will come after. Dr. Martin Luther King Jr. was one who came before. Dr. King was "someone able to admit how often he was afraid and unsure about his next step…It was his human vulnerability and his ability to rise above it that I most remember. He did not pretend to be a great powerful know-it-all. I remember him discussing openly his gloom, depression, his fears, admitting that he did not know what the next step was. He would then say: "Take the first step in faith. You don't have to see the whole staircase, just take the first step" (Marian Wright Edelman, founder of the Children's Defense Fund as quoted by Loeb, 2010, p. 57). My students will take these steps as so many will after.

Our work is powerful, poignant, personal, professional, and political. As written earlier, I grew up impacted by the 1960s and 1970s. Those were times of change where there were critical movements furthering social justice. There were social activists and peace activists such as Martin Luther King, Jr., John F. Kennedy, and Malcolm X, among others, that led revolutions of progressive change. In March 1968, during his "Remaining Awake Through a Great Revolution" speech at the National Cathedral Dr. Martin Luther King Jr. said, "We shall overcome because the arc of the moral universe is long but it bends towards justice."

Author's Note I want to specially acknowledge Connie Baechler for her thoughtful comments and support through the completion of this chapter. Your support has been very special to me while "looking into the mirror."

References

Bell, L. A., Griffin, P., & Adams, M. (Eds.). (2007). *Teaching for diversity and social justice.* Routledge: New York.

Comas-Díaz, L., & Torres Rivera, E. (Eds.). (2020). *Liberation psychology: Theory, method, practice, and social justice.* American Psychological Association.

Loeb, P. R. (2010). *Soul of a citizen: Living with conviction in challenging times*. St. Martin's Publishing Group.

Mock, M. (2019). Social justice in family therapy training: The power of personal and family narratives. In K. V. Hardy & M. McGoldrick (Eds.), *Re-visioning family therapy: Addressing diversity in clinical practice* (pp. 496–511). Guilford Publications.

On Being Influenced: How an Alumni of Color Scholarship Program Invites Diverse Voices into Program Leadership

Elisabeth Esmiol Wilson

In my practice as a sex therapist, I have begun to regularly ask my clients to experiment with what Dr. Kerner (2021) calls Willingness-Windows. These are moments when folks in relationship set aside time to show up with the willingness to "have a vulnerable conversation" or "be pushed out of your comfort zone in a way that's important to your sexual development" (p. 293). I remember a session with a couple who immediately liked the idea of Willingness-Windows, but when I saw them the next week, the wife shared "I think that was much harder than either of us expected. I think we were scared." This couple was simultaneously experiencing both desire and fear, wanting to meet each other with defenses down, yet terrified of truly opening to their own and the other's vulnerability. In therapy, I am most passionate about this tension between fear and desire, and helping clients lean into these emotions as the pathway to deeper connection. In teaching, I am equally passionate about supporting my graduate students in learning to choreograph such vulnerable encounters, where the "internal drama moves into the interpersonal realm" and people in relationships truly sense and see each other (Johnson, 2019, p. 61). Facilitating my second year Couple/Marriage and Family Therapy (C/MFT) graduate students in guiding and structuring these intimate moments in relationship and sex counseling brings me great joy. However, I found a place in my own work as a professor and especially as director of clinical training, where I began to notice that familiar mixture of fear and desire in myself. This place inside myself had everything to do with my own intersecting identities as a white, heterosexual, cis gender female tenured faculty member. Specifically, I found myself feeling both desire and fear around my own willingness to be significantly influenced by diverse voices to make meaningful changes as a leader.

E. E. Wilson (✉)
Pacific Lutheran University, Tacoma, WA, USA

NW Reflections Counseling, Puyallup, WA, USA

© American Family Therapy Academy (AFTA) 2023
L. A. Nice, C. Eppler (eds.), *Social Justice and Systemic Family Therapy Training*,
AFTA SpringerBriefs in Family Therapy, https://doi.org/10.1007/978-3-031-29930-8_5

1   Context and Identities

I had been teaching for nearly a decade in a small, predominantly white C/MFT department in the politically liberal Pacific Northwest at a historically white university that was becoming increasingly centered on social justice. However, I was collecting important feedback from our graduate students and alumni about the lack of contextually informed, culturally sensitive clinical training folks were receiving. At the time, almost half of our practicum students reported that their supervisors were not facilitating conversations about clients' intersecting identities as part of clinical supervision. As the Director of Clinical Training (DCT), I had significant work to do to move our clinical training program toward becoming more anti-racist, anti-homophobic, and anti-sexist. I identify as white: a descendant of more recent German immigrants as well as early British colonists. I am a cis gender, AFAB (assigned female at birth), heterosexual, middle aged wife, mother, stepmom, and a recent grandmother. I have a large extended family in New England, but was born in Hawaii where I grew up with my single mother actively participating in our LGBTQ affirming, multi-racial Episcopal church on Oahu. After graduating from a predominantly Asian high school in Hawaii, I spent 12 years in higher education, graduating from Harvard College, earning a Master of Arts as a Spiritual Director, finding my professional home as a C/MFT with a masters and doctorate, then becoming an American Association of Marriage and Family Therapy (AAMFT) approved supervisor and an American Association of Sexuality Educatory, Counselors and Therapists (AASECT) certified sex therapist. With my background and specific intersecting identities, I hold a lot of privilege, and I felt both excited and scared to help lead the way toward a more socially just clinical training program. At times my internal voice seemed to scream: *You're not the one for this job. Just quit and hire a person with more marginalized identities. You're making too many mistakes that you often don't even see!* But I also heard that part of me desiring change and a program where all students, alumni, and clients felt a sense of inclusion and belonging. Sometimes just a whisper, that voice replied: *There needs to be a change. Use your privilege for good. Lead by example, repairing mistakes visibly.*

2   Launching an Alumni of Color Scholarship Program

In this context of awareness about needing to become more anti-racist, anti-homophobic, and anti-sexist, and alongside department changes led by our program director, I helped initiate a new scholarship designed to increase the number of supervisors of Color in our clinical training program and our state. Initially, if I am fully transparent, I was not aware that this scholarship program was also going to invite diverse voices into our program leadership. Only over time would I be confronted with the mix of my own fears and desires around staying open and influenceable to these voices calling for change. At the beginning, the new program seemed simple enough: any alumni of Color from our program with 2 years post licensure could apply for the scholarship and the department would pay all the AAMFT Supervision Training fees including supervision of supervision as well as pay the alumni recipient to supervise up to two of our practicum students in our onsite university clinic. We contracted out the supervision of supervision, hiring a C/MFT of Color with decades of experience, and launched our scholarship program.

3 Early Lessons and Awareness of Privilege

3.1 Prioritizing Supervisor Choice and Relationships

One of the early lessons we learned was that just because a supervisor in training and their supervisor of supervision are both folks of Color does not mean that the working relationship will be supportive. This may seem obvious, but it helped us prioritize choice and relationships over sharing particular identities. We began to support our scholarship recipients in choosing their own supervisor of supervision from a select group of folks we worked with, including the faculty. While I never imagined myself, as a white woman, providing supervision of supervision to any of our alumni of Color, I found myself at times in just that position. And to my great surprise, even after folks earned their AAMFT Approved Supervisor status, some stayed in the supervision of supervision group with me, co-facilitating and supporting newer supervisors-in-training.

3.2 Centering Experiences of Racism

Another early lesson I realized, as the only white woman in a group of supervisors of Color, was the depth of support necessary for continuing to work interracially and the importance of collectively holding space to process experiences of ongoing racism and homophobia. I have participated in many supervision and consultation groups over the years. Sometimes these groups have been all white, and sometimes they have included one or two therapists of Color. This was my first experience as the only white therapist in a group, made more pronounced by my leadership role as the Approved Supervisor, and what stood out to me was the ability of group members to center their experiences of racism in our conversations. In one group session, a queer Indigenous member was in tears sharing a traumatizing experience of seeing a white police officer accost a homeless person of Color outside their office window as they were providing online supervision to a student therapist. As I took a one-down position, the supervisors-in-training supported this group member in processing their anger and grief, highlighting how this person was able to center themselves, name the impact and injustice of overt racism, and lean on resources including relationships with each other.

3.3 Directly Addressing Racism and Sexism at All Levels

One more early lesson we learned was that students, and not just white students, held internalized biases against learning from supervisors of Color, and supervisors of Color with additional intersecting marginalized identities that included being female, queer, a non-native English speaker, or of a non-Christian religious background, that needed to be addressed directly. Unfortunately, I have more examples than I ever imagined of students dismissing the clinical feedback from our new scholarship recipients who joined us as supervisors-in-training. Again in full transparency, I at first tried to explain away the embedded racism in this dynamic by suggesting that perhaps students were reacting to the fact that their supervisor was in training. However, we had white supervisors-in-training at off-site clinics that were not receiving this dismissive and disrespectful treatment. When a white male student ignored his Latina supervisor's clinical advice and later phoned another white male supervisor for his advice, our supervision of supervision group processed how the male supervisor redirecting the student therapist back to his Latina supervisor was not enough. I had to face my own white discomfort around overtly naming the racism and not colluding with this white male supervisor in feeling it was enough to simply redirect the male student back to his supervisor of Color. Only by directly naming the dynamic for what it was, both racist and sexist, with everyone involved, were we able to make any change. The supervisor of Color named the racism and sexism with the white male student in supervision, inviting him to reflect on his internalized biases and supporting him in beginning to take ownership for his impact not just on her but on potential clients of Color. We also met together with the white male supervisor and named the racism I was tempted to be complicit with, and highlighted how he needed to not just redirect the student but directly name the implicit racism and sexism. Finally his Latina supervisor together with myself and another white faculty member met with the white male student to further process his ongoing deconstruction of internalized racism and support his commitment to culturally sensitive treatment of supervisors and clients of Color.

3.4 Empowering Supervisor Growth Through Mentorship

Another important lesson we learned was how to better support supervisor growth through mentorship. Some of our alumni of Color had graduated as many as 10 years before returning as clinical supervisors-in-training. In addition to processing personal and professional experiences of racism and countering students' implicit racial biases, these new supervisors also were figuring out new policies in our university clinic, navigating a new world of supervision via telehealth, and learning how to be supervisors for the first time. What we found was that our supervisors-in-training benefited from a mentorship program where they partnered with another AAMFT Approved supervisor and did co-supervision for one semester before working on their own. Again we supported our scholarship recipients in choosing the Approved Supervisor they wanted to partner with, and then supported the Approved Supervisor in mentoring, co-leading, and eventually, by the end of the semester, taking a one-down position as the supervisor-in-training primarily led supervision. This model has proved much more supportive of supervisor growth. However, additional dynamics of power and privilege emerged, especially for supervisors of Color who partnered with white Approved Supervisors, as I will describe in the following text.

4 Repairing Relational Ruptures

I have come to deeply appreciate these moments of rupture and repair as the heart of my work as a therapist, professor, supervisor, and most basically as a human being. Over the years I have learned to gather up and treasure these stories of relational repair. I have many of them in many different contexts, but the moments I seem to learn the most from are the ones where I am at the center of unintentionally causing the hurt. Through much self-reflection on such moments, I have come to hold the following four aspects of repair as essential: (1) not being shocked at myself for making a mistake and giving myself grace for being human (which prevents becoming defensive or going into a shame spiral); (2) staying open and listening deeply to the other person's experience and feedback; (3) taking responsibility by directly naming my wrong and the impact I had on the other; (4) genuinely extending care with an open heart to what the other person needs. Practicing and modeling these four aspects of repair are a core part of what it means to be an influenceable leader.

4.1 Repair Number One

Following our mentorship model, I had the honor of co-facilitating a practicum group with a Chinese American cis gender female supervisor-in-training, who I will refer to by the pseudonym Fen. Our supervision group consisted of four white, cis gender female therapists, two of whom identified as queer, and one as polyamorous. During our semester together, we experienced two significant moments of processing rupture and repair. The first moment occurred near the beginning of the semester after Fen and I completed our second co-supervision session together. We had decided to meet for 30 min after each weekly supervision session to debrief together. During this particular supervision debriefing session, we began with me checking in on our co-supervision relationship. It is important to note that Fen had actually been a former student of mine and one of my earliest supervisees.

Elisabeth: I wanted to start today and check in with you about how you felt we did today collaborating and co-leading?

Fen: I was glad you started the session so I could see how you checked in with each person. And I didn't know some of their documentation and clinic-specific questions, so that was helpful having you answer those. I felt a little nervous when you handed over some of the clinical supervision to me but I liked stepping in and helping students with their cases.

Elisabeth: I really appreciated how you helped Angel with her biracial couples case. The questions you offered her to help discuss the impact of their racial and cultural differences really seemed to not just help her but also the other students.

Fen: Thanks. It felt good to hear their feedback that I was helping them, and it also felt like here I am, the one non-white therapist in the room, and the only one really pointing out that the couple's cultural differences needed to be integrated into their therapy.

At this point I felt myself feeling embarrassed and also a bit defensive thinking that I would have also asked Angel about the couple's cultural differences if I wasn't trying to give Fen space to supervise. However, the point was that Fen had been the one to address their racial identities first, and the impact on her was negative.

Elisabeth: That's true, you were the first one to highlight their cultural differences. I imagine as the only person of color in the group that felt like either no one else noticed their differences or were waiting for you to do the work of noticing.

Fen: I kind of felt that way when I was a student here too.

I really felt my stomach sink at this point. I intuitively knew I had to not only address her experience as a former student in our department, but specifically her experience with me as her former supervisor. I imagined what the relational and clinical impact had been on her of having me as her supervisor almost a decade ago. I had been a young white professor new to teaching and supervising and certainly even less aware at the time of directly integrating racial identities into treatment.

Elisabeth: Fen, I am so sorry. It is especially not the responsibility of a student to feel they need to bring up cultural issues in supervision. I'm wondering if you'd like to process your experience of supervision with me when you were a student here with me?

Fen: I think that'd be helpful.

Elisabeth: Would you like to share first or have me share first?

Fen: You can start.

Elisabeth: I never told you this as a student, and thinking about it today, it may have helped if I had told you. But at the time, I think I felt embarrassed that I wasn't doing a good job. I knew I wasn't understanding you or how you were doing therapy but I didn't name the cultural gap between us, a white female supervisor and a Chinese American therapist. I actually consulted with an older supervisor of Color who eventually became a mentor of mine. She was helpful in slowing me down and noticing how you were practicing therapy out of your intersecting identities. But I don't think I ever communicated this effectively to you, and I imagine you felt like I didn't see you or understand you in supervision.

Fen: I didn't feel supported in the program or in supervision with you. It was really hard feeling like I didn't belong in the clinic and I didn't see anyone who looked like me doing therapy like me. I spent a long time even after graduation doubting myself. I really struggled to even accept this scholarship, but I knew I wanted to help other students of Color not feel the way I did back then.

Elisabeth: I know I didn't provide what you needed and I really want to try to make this experience of working together again different – as much as I can.

Fen: It feels really different just talking about this. I'm in a different place today. And I'm glad you recognize you weren't there for me.

Elisabeth: As hard as it is, I hold our supervision experience as a reminder of how much I want to work at directly naming differences and making space to talk about intersecting identities.

Fen: Yeah, I saw that last week. It felt really different in our first co-supervision group when we all introduced ourselves and you asked us to talk about our different intersecting identities and the identities most important to us. I wasn't sure at first if you would have done that if I wasn't there. But it was nice hearing students share that they've done this before and liked learning new things about each other each time they reintroduced themselves. It's sort of amazing to be back and feel like maybe some of the hurt can finally start to heal.

4.2   Repair Number Two

This conversation felt like the beginning of that healing process for Fen with me, and also within the program at large. Her voice would grow to be one of the diverse voices that would lead to significant program changes. But there was still one more important moment of rupture and repair from later that semester worth sharing. Our supervision group included four white cis women: Angel, who identified as polyamorous, Sue and Sami, who identified as queer, and Kat, who identified as heterosexual (all pseudonyms). Over halfway through the semester, an Asian hate crime occurred in a nearby city which received both news and social media coverage. At the start of our next group supervision 3 days after the hate crime, I began with our typical opening of inviting everyone to start with a check in. I did not bring up the tragedy of the hate crime. Angel, Sue, Sami, and Kat all shared, none of them mentioning the Asian hate crime. Sometimes after the students shared, Fen and I would briefly share a check in.

Angel: Fen or Elisabeth, do you want to check in today too?

Fen: Sure. I can share briefly. It's been a really hard few days for me with the news.

Elisabeth: [I paused and waited. When Fen didn't say more I felt that she didn't want to process her feelings with the supervision group. I made note to check in with her during our post supervision debrief.] Thanks Fen for letting us know. I'm doing ok today. Let's move to discussing cases. Who wants to share first?

After our supervision session Fen and I met for half an hour and I asked her how she was doing in processing the recent hate crimes. We talked about how she was reaching out to resources in her family and community. We discussed a couple of student cases and planned on checking in next time with Kat who seemed hesitant about bringing up cases in group. The next day, shortly before our supervision of supervision group, Fen forwarded me an email from Angel and Sami:

Email: Dear Fen, We want to apologize that we didn't ask you how you were doing. After you shared, we felt really uncomfortable that Elisabeth moved us directly to cases without inviting you to process and share more. We didn't speak up and felt like we were dismissing you and your pain. We apologize for this microaggression and not being more sensitive in supervision. Please let us know if you want to talk about this with us. Sincerely, Angel and Sami.

On reading the email I immediately saw how my not checking in with Fen during our supervision group was a microaggression. I already knew from our debrief that I had read her correctly, but I also was aware that if I had been wrong, the impact could have been very hurtful. At the beginning of supervision, I checked in with Fen to see if she was open to processing the email and my response in our group with me and the other supervisors of Color.

Fen: Yes, I do want to process the email. [She read the email to the group.] I was honestly surprised to receive their email. I'm touched that they were really sensitive to how I was doing even though I really didn't want to discuss it in group with them.

Elisabeth: How does it fit for you to think of me not checking in with you as a microaggression?

Fen: I don't think I would have thought of that. Really, if I'd wanted to say more, I would have.

Elisabeth: And while I also made the assumption that you would say more if you wanted to, I appreciate the students noticing that I didn't ask you. And what if I was wrong, and in that moment you needed to be invited to share more, especially as the only Asian American in the room, and as the supervisor-in-training.

Fen: I guess I hadn't thought about it that way. But yeah, I can see how that could be a microaggression and how it'd be nice to be the one to say "I'm done talking, your turn Elisabeth."

We continued to process this rupture of a microaggression with the other supervisors of Color and planned on addressing Angel and Sami's email with our supervision group next week. Fen led the discussion the following week, shared her experience of our last supervision group, and then I took ownership, acknowledged that my making an assumption about Fen was a microaggression, and thanked Angel and Sami for bringing this to our attention. Fen followed up by sharing how healing co-leading this supervision group had been for her by working with students who were so aware and sensitive to her cultural context.

4.3 Reflections on Relational Repair

Early on, repairing with one person was hard enough for me without an "audience." However, I also know that we learn in the context of relationships, that relational ruptures need relational repair, and that repair can actually deepen attachment security (Fishbane, 2007; Makinen & Johnson, 2006; Tronick, 1989). Today, I treasure such moments of repair, like with Fen, and share them regularly and transparently in class and supervision, modeling possible pathways for repair through my own mistakes. As demonstrated in the first repair attempt in the preceding text, we can hold both hurts and the possibility for healing even after many, many years. The second example of repair shows some growth in how I try to model repair attempts in real time and collectively. Processing my microaggression alone with Fen would have been a missed opportunity that deepened our understanding of repair as we shared this experience in our supervision of supervision group. Because my mistake happened in Fen's and my supervision group, processing the repair collectively with Angel, Sami, Kat, and Sue was essential. I also have learned that modeling repair for racial ruptures, while absolutely necessary, is not sufficient for being a contextually sensitive leader.

5 Beyond Anti-racist Policy to Follow Through

Simply stated, repair without follow through and new action does not create lasting change. The depth of this truth became apparent to me through staying open to the influence of our Supervisors of Color. Sometimes a moment of relational rupture simply needs to be addressed directly, but at other times, policy must be followed or created to prevent continued damage. One of the huge benefits of our mentorship model of co-leading supervision groups and then processing with other Supervisors of Color in our supervision of supervision group was a more collaborative model of discussing and following through on policy issues. Over the years of our scholarship program we had several student issues arise that in the past would have led to extra student meetings or a note in the student's file. However, one of the places where I found myself significantly opening up to being influenced by the leadership of our Supervisors of Color was in recognizing important ways I had not enforced our policy, to the detriment of student learning and our program's well-being. The following example shows the overall benefit to students and the clinical program of intentionally and thoroughly following through on anti-racist clinical training policy.

5.1   Holding Students Accountable

Every semester, supervisors complete a clinical competency evaluation for each student in clinical practicum. One of the competency expectations is that a student therapist "initiates dialogue and demonstrates sensitivity regarding contextual consciousness throughout the session." What we found through live and video observation was that particularly white students with more privilege were not *initiating* clinical conversations about race. An important step toward anti-racist policy follow through for me occurred in supervision of supervision as we discussed the impact (or lack of impact) of simply marking students "below expected" on this particular competency, semester after semester. At the time, supervision of supervision consisted of Kalisha, a multi-racial Black cis female heterosexual supervisor, Chenoa, an Indigenous cis female heterosexual supervisor, and Mariana, a Latina non-binary, queer supervisor. We were near the end of the semester and discussing two white, cis gender, heterosexual students likely to receive "below expected" for the contextual consciousness competency: Daniel, an intern in his first practicum supervised by Kalisha, and Summer, an intern in her last practicum supervised by Chenoa. Chenoa had just informed us that in her last live supervision of a new intake with a multiracial couple, Summer did not initiate dialogue about intersecting identities.

Elisabeth: It sounds like Summer is still not meeting this competency, and is likely going to receive "below expected" yet again.

Chenoa: We say that contextual consciousness and culturally sensitive therapy is one of our core program learning outcomes. Yet it sounds like it's possible for a student to graduate without ever demonstrating this competency. I'm curious, what's the point of "below expected?"

These moments of realization, highlighting patterns of white privilege that perpetuate an unacceptable level of clinical incompetence, are painful. Noticing my own pain internally helps me catch myself from either becoming defensive or going down a shame spiral. I internally held my pain with gentle hands and recognized this moment as an opportunity for change.

Elisabeth: Wow. It feels really obvious as you say that, Chenoa, that you're right. What we've been doing so far really isn't helping Summer become a better therapist.

Chenoa: It just seems like we're repeating last semester. Despite my conversations with Summer in supervision about her needing to initiate conversations about race with her clients, I didn't see change. I gave her "below expected" at the end of the semester; then you and the other core faculty met with her together. And yet I'm not seeing the necessary change now in her last semester.

Kalisha: I wonder what would be different for Summer if after receiving "below expected" she met with me, a Black woman, and with you Chenoa, an Indigenous woman, and with Mariana, a queer Latina, instead of with an all-white faculty? I just question how much she's really feeling challenged.

Mariana: I hear you Kalisha, and I also don't know if it's just talking with white faculty versus supervisors of Color. I think it goes beyond that to actually having and following through with anti-racist policy. Elisabeth, do we have policies that could help us require some significant changes for Summer? Could we hold her back from graduating in a few months to repeat a practicum?

I honestly had to pause at this point. I appreciated the nuance Mariana made around Kalisha's question: highlighting that the real question, beyond our different intersecting identities, was "How are we being anti-racist in our leadership?" I also had to admit that, yes, we had policies in place to prevent a student from passing practicum or require a student to take an additional semester of practicum if not meeting a core clinical competency. And, if I was honest with myself, our faculty had failed former students for not meeting competencies around ethical issues of confidentiality and paperwork, but never for ethical issues of contextual consciousness. Again I held my emotions with gentle hands and leaned into transparency and accountability.

Elisabeth: Thank you for these necessary and challenging questions. Yes, we have policies in place to require Summer to take another practicum. I need to own my own lack of leadership in following through with our policies, especially in this area of cultural competence. And that's not okay, and needs to change.

5.2   High Standards Benefit All

We spent time discussing the specific policy follow through that would most benefit Summer. We also talked about the benefit not just to Summer and her clients, but to current students in the program watching Summer's sessions, and to future students who will enter a program actually upholding rigorous standards for contextually conscious, culturally sensitive practice. In the end, both Summer and Daniel repeated practicum along with written, reading, and process-based requirements to examine their implicit biases and increase anti-racist practices. These requirements eventually became mandatory for all students with privileged identities, through the format of a monthly process group. We experienced many unexpected benefits as a result of having a required cross-cohort space where more privileged students were facilitated by alumni of our program in processing their internal racial biases without a supervisor or faculty member and without being graded. As we began to follow through with our anti-racist policies, we initially saw several students repeating practicum, though in time those numbers decreased.

6   Recommendations and Takeaways for Programmatic Change

Collectively as a department, in collaboration with our Supervisors of Color, and in my leadership role as the Director of Clinical Training, we are still growing, learning, repairing ruptures, gathering feedback, making mistakes, and making improvements in becoming more inclusive and socially just. Transitioning toward an anti-racist, anti-homophobic, and anti-sexist clinical training program often feels messy, at times overwhelming and exhausting, and simultaneously moving to be involved in such intentional healing and change. In conclusion, I tentatively offer a brief list of recommendations for replicating similar programmatic change. I want to honor that every program is unique and the changes needed depend on the specific compilation of faculty, supervisors, students, and the populations of clients served. Honoring the uniqueness of each program, I offer the following takeaways that have helped guide us in the hopes that some may be useful to others.

6.1 Assessment and Feedback

At the heart of our commitment to staying open to influence, we deliberately and intentionally created a culture of bi-directional feedback. As faculty and as supervisors, we supported each other in remaining accountable to not only providing regular and specific feedback, but also giving students and supervisees regular opportunities to provide both verbal and written feedback to us. We supported students in using this bi-directional model with their clients, requiring the regular use of written client feedback at the end of every session.

6.2 Listening to Diverse Voices by Challenging Dominant Perspectives

For our specific program, centering diverse voices was only possible after first taking accountability for the historic legacy of being part of predominantly white, male institutions embedded with patriarchal, misogynistic, racist, homophobic practices. Only then were we able to understand how dominant culture values impacted our own training and teaching. We took responsibility for pursuing our own development in deconstructing privilege and all the discriminatory ideologies. We also challenged dominant perspectives by increasingly centering the different voices, perspectives, values, and beliefs of our supervisors of Color to help expand contextually aware, socially just practices (Scarborough, 2017).

6.3 Becoming Influenceable Leaders Through Awareness of Impact

How, in our privilege, do we strive to become an ally, and learn to be aware of the invisible, that is, microaggressions, and dominant cultural dynamics? Part of becoming an influenceable leader involves letting go of "being right" or even "getting it right" and learning to be aware of our impact. We notice our impact on others to the degree that we can set aside the need to prove or defend our good intentions, and instead privilege the experience of the other.

6.4 Policy in Action: Addressing Racism and Deconstructing Privilege

Some of the examples in this chapter highlighted specific moments in our program where we honestly confronted how we were not following through and putting policy into action. First we must undergo the hard work of reviewing and rewriting our programmatic policies. However, even socially just policies are only helpful to the degree that we put policy into action through continuously and actively naming and rejecting the influence of dominant, oppressive discourses.

6.5 Empowering Marginalized Community Members

How do we as leaders empower marginalized community members? This journey involves learning to collaborate not dominate, to embrace diversity not sameness, to engage relationally not hierarchically. It may be helpful to ponder: to what degree am I open to valuing different sources of knowledge, different research methods, different structures of leadership, different decision-making processes? True empowerment comes as we recognize our need for each other.

6.6 Creating a Culture Care, an Ethics of Care, a Politics of Care

Early in the development of our program we were excited to build a culture of feedback, and our commitment to being open to student feedback, integrating suggestions from graduates, and willing to collaborate and make changes was a huge strength. However, openness to feedback alone was not enough. As we began making changes, we found that we had to care for ourselves as leaders, both faculty and supervisors, modeling boundaries and creating enough margin for rest, and then modeling this for students and building in such margin in our curriculum, assignments, and clinical caseloads for students. However, caring for ourselves and our students was also not enough. We realized we had to foster a culture of care for our clients that went beyond clinical compassion toward an ethics of care and a politics of care that challenges the very economic and political systems perpetuating oppression (Watson et al., 2020).

6.7 Diverse Voices Throughout Curriculum

As educators, we must commit to regularly and rigorously revising and expanding our curriculum to include new perspectives. To do this we must move beyond our professionally siloed networks and engage across disciplines as well as outside of traditionally academic structures. We must embrace a willingness to disrupt the status quo by truly allowing ourselves to be radically influenced.

References

Fishbane, M. D. (2007). Wired to connect: Neuroscience, relationships, and therapy. *Family Process, 46*(3), 395–412. https://doi.org/10.1111/j.1545-5300.2007.00219.x

Johnson, S. M. (2019). *Attachment theory in practice: Emotionally focused therapy (EFT) with individuals, couples, and families.* Guilford Publications.

Kerner, I. (2021). *So tell me about the last time you had sex: Laying bare and learning to repair our love lives.* Grand Central Publishing.

Makinen, J. A., & Johnson, S. M. (2006). Resolving attachment injuries in couples using emotionally focused therapy: Steps toward forgiveness and reconciliation. *Journal of Consulting and Clinical Psychology, 74*(6), 1055–1064. https://doi.org/10.1037/0022-006X.74.6.1055

Scarborough, N. (2017). When dominant culture values meet diverse clinical settings: Perspectives from an African American supervisor. In R. Allen & S. S. Poulsen (Eds.), *Creating culture safety in couple and family therapy: Supervision and training* (AFTA Springer Briefs). Springer.

Tronick, E. Z. (1989). Emotions and emotional communication in infants. *The American Psychologist, 44*(2), 112–119. https://doi.org/10.1037//0003-066x.44.2.112

Watson, M. F., Bacigalupe, G., Daneshpour, M., Han, W. J., & Parra-Cardona, R. (2020). COVID-19 Interconnectedness: Health Inequity, the Climate Crisis, and Collective Trauma. *Family process, 59*(3), 832–846. https://doi.org/10.1111/famp.12572

Addressing Issues of Race on Campus in a Couple and Family Therapy Graduate Program

Jennifer M. Sampson

Before I begin, it is important to locate myself in position to you, the reader. I am a mixed-race, light-skinned, Filipino cis-woman. I am also a queer person married to a White, cis-hetero-man. I largely benefit from having an able-body but I struggle with some invisible disabilities, including hearing challenges and infertility. I recently became a mother to a healthy mixed-race child – one who has inherited the Nordic skin qualities of both of his parents, along with his father's blue eyes. Even just a few months in, it is easy to see that it is not likely that his Filipino heritage will be visibly obvious to anyone looking at him. When I let myself stop to think about it, I feel a burden of responsibility to teach him how to be responsible with all of the privilege he has coming his way.

I grew up in a home with two married parents in North Dakota – the land of freezing temperatures and conservative values. My father was born and raised there, and my mother was an immigrant from the Philippines, here on a work visa working as a nurse when she met my father on his medical school surgical rotation. Our family was financially privileged, and I attended Catholic schools for 13 years. While I have left Catholicism and the Midwest far behind, the narratives from having grown up in those contexts have frontloaded my life with plenty of biases in need of unpacking.

I found my way to the West Coast for graduate school and became a couple and family therapist (CFT). Even after 6 years of higher education, I believe that my real learning began when I was accepted into a Minority Fellowship Program during my doctoral program. I was connected with a group of Black, Indigenous, and People of Color (BIPOC) peers whose conversations and influence forced me to turn inward and start critically looking at myself and my own biases, privilege, and areas where

J. M. Sampson (✉)
Antioch University, Seattle, WA, USA
e-mail: jsampson1@antioch.edu

© American Family Therapy Academy (AFTA) 2023
L. A. Nice, C. Eppler (eds.), *Social Justice and Systemic Family Therapy Training*,
AFTA SpringerBriefs in Family Therapy, https://doi.org/10.1007/978-3-031-29930-8_6

I have experienced oppression, in ways I had never been required to do in any previous setting. Since then, I have had to unlearn a lot of things that my upbringing and my professional training taught me, and through that, I have come to understand this about myself – that I am an ambiguous mix of privileged and oppressed parts, and I often struggle with how to reconcile them. And I have come to be okay with that.

Now as the leader of a CFT graduate program in the Pacific Northwest, I have the privilege of guiding a team of faculty and students toward doing the most challenging and, what I believe to be, the most important work of our lives – learning about power and privilege and how to navigate that in a way that creates space, love, and respect for everyone.

1 Introduction

Following the murder of George Floyd, the members of the Black Student Union (BSU) on our campus came together and delivered a letter to campus administration, titled "Hear Our Voices" (BSU, 2020). The letter contained a list of concerns, demands, and requests directly addressing institutional racism that they and other BIPOC students had experienced during their time in their academic programs. The students described examples of disparate treatment of Black students at all levels of their university experience, from peers in and outside of the classrooms to interactions with the faculty and staff during the admissions process and in using student services. The letter also included the results of a survey of Black students on our campus that found that during their time at the university:

- 83% of participants had experienced microaggressions
- 33% of participants had experienced explicit racial discrimination
- 67% of participants had felt unsafe in the classroom
- 17% of participants had felt isolation.

These findings are backed in the literature. As racial diversity in higher education institutions increases, there has been a greater increase in racial tensions, manifesting through microaggressions, discrimination, threats, and even violence (Stotzer & Hossellman, 2012). A 2000study on campus racial climate by Solórzano, Ceja, and Yosso found that when Black students experienced racial microaggressions, including verbal and nonverbal attacks, they felt academically and socially isolated.

Furthermore, the BSU letter included a list of demands – like the development of a plan of action in collaboration with Black students to address racial inequity and lack of inclusion – as well as requests – such as additional funding opportunities for BIPOC students and an update to campus evaluations to include an assessment of faculty, staff, and administration's attention to diversity issues at various levels of the system.

In the following weeks, our program faculty assembled with the objective to take a hard look at how our program is structured and what changes we can make to place anti-racism at the heart of our program. This chapter summarizes some of the things we did in our program to directly confront institutional racism in our system. I will describe some of our processes, ideas, setbacks, and failures in the hope that some of our work may be helpful to you.

2 Redefining Our Program's Mission

One of the very first changes our CFT faculty put into place was the adaptation of our mission statement and the creation of a vision statement that could be used to guide the work and decisions in our program. We joined together in one of our faculty meetings and made a collective decision to amend our mission statement to directly state that we are focused on centering anti-oppressive teaching in our program. This was generally accepted by the faculty with some pushback from one of our program's leaders, but despite this, over the upcoming weeks we workshopped language for these updates that the majority of the faculty in our program felt captured the spirit and direction that we wanted our program to take.

Mission statement: *The mission of [our] program is to prepare and train knowledgeable, skilled, self-aware, ethical, and anti-racist couple and family therapists in a learning environment that centers anti-white supremacy and social justice in its academic experience.*

Values statement: [Our] *program supports anti-racist and anti-oppressive practices by confronting and rejecting white supremacy and systemic inequality through socially just and systemically oriented academic instruction. We will take an active stance against white supremacy, marginalization, dehumanization, and systemic oppression while teaching our students to engage in active resistance and advocacy in their work as individual, relationship, couple, and family therapists. We value self-awareness and cultural responsiveness of our faculty, students, and graduates and strive to create opportunities for these personal learning processes to happen across systemic levels.*

From there, we established a set of guiding principles from which we would work in developing our new anti-racist processes. These principles focused on centering voices of People of Color (faculty members, students, and staff), rather than white voices in decision-making and conversations.

Once our conversations shifted toward strategies for centering the voices of People of Color, dynamics began to shift among faculty. For example, a white faculty member who raised mild concerns about the shift in mission statement became even more vocal about their concerns about the changes that explicitly decentered White voices. This – unsurprisingly – was not well-received by the other faculty members, especially the faculty members of color. While the changes we made to our mission and faculty expectations were accepted by the campus and university administration, it did start the process of creating fractures in faculty relationships with one another.

3   Faculty Development Efforts

From there, we took a look at our faculty. We wanted to consider and recognize how our faculty members may have been contributing to oppressive systems at our university. The letter from the Black Student Union described that only 37% of Black students who completed their survey indicated that faculty "actively create safe spaces by countering harmful anti-Black stereotypes if and when it occurs in the classroom"; 25% reported that they felt faculty did not do this at all. These numbers did not sit well with us.

3.1   Recruitment and Retention of BIPOC Faculty Members

At this point in time, only five of our fourteen faculty members were people of Color. In order to truly center BIPOC voices, we knew we needed to do better about representing them on our faculty. We established a hiring committee that was tasked with reviewing and developing faculty hiring strategies that were aimed at recruiting and retaining faculty members of Color. We also doubled down on our efforts to recruit more faculty of Color for adjunct positions as well.

Recruitment and retention of faculty members of Color is a challenge in higher education across the country for a variety of reasons, including overlooked unique emotional burden experienced by faculty with marginalized identities when faced with challenges of confronting the unspoken normative principles of whiteness in academic institutions (Hayes & Juárez, 2009; Turner, 2002). In an effort to address these issues in our processing, our hiring committee engaged strategies including ensuring BIPOC representation on hiring committees, including BIPOC student representation, curating job descriptions, postings, and interview processes to attract applicants of Color as well as those who prioritize and value anti-racism and anti-oppression work in their teaching.

We found that focusing on these things during the recruitment process allowed for applicants to get a sense of what our program was about and also prepare them for our students who take their roles as "therapist as activist" seriously in the classroom. Through the interview process we were able to better differentiate those who had a more integrated value of anti-racism work versus those who may have less experience doing so.

Various faculty members experienced personal challenges with these changes in the process, reflecting that their own interview experience did not focus on anti-racism in a similar way. These shifts brought to the surface insecurities from various faculty and staff about whether or not they were doing a "good enough" job at upholding these new standards themselves, and this anxiety influenced dynamics in a variety of ways, from willingness to participate in conversations to rejection of certain decisions being made among the faculty.

3.2   Standardizing Classroom Expectations

We developed a workgroup that was tasked with standardizing faculty expectations for centering anti-racism and anti-oppression in the classroom and in interactions with students. This group, co-facilitated by BIPOC and white faculty members, came up with the expectations of the CFT faculty members, which included providing faculty trainings and processes about handling challenging conversations centered around race, including use of small caucus groups in the classroom; utilization of land acknowledgements and emotional labor statements in each syllabus; asking faculty to socially locate themselves with their students each quarter; and diversifying course materials to center the work of BIPOC authors, researchers, scholars, and artists.

3.3   Faculty Evaluations

In an effort to monitor and assess how our faculty were doing at following through with these commitments, we reviewed and integrated diversity competencies into faculty evaluations. We added items for students to rate their instructors on their inclusion of course materials that represent contextually diverse perspectives and also the instructors' inclusion of classroom discussions regarding diverse perspectives and experiences. Additionally, the end of year faculty evaluation process includes a required self-evaluation reflecting on what it means to them to be a faculty member in the context of the University's commitment to being an anti-racist institution.

3.4   Communication with Students

We co-authored a written statement explicitly rejecting racial supremacy, anti-Blackness, and the hate-filled racist ideology of intolerance that is used to oppress People of Color. We stated our commitment to driving forward for as long as it takes to force systemic change in our institution and in our CFT field. We committed to engaging in open dialogue around important policy and systemic issues, in an effort to make radical changes to laws that continue to perpetuate destructive patterns in our country.

Alongside this, we took a look at our relationships with our students – particularly our Students of Color. In order to examine this more closely, our program reached out to the Black Student Union and the Counselors of Color Student Support Groups on campus to develop a process for dialogue and feedback. We met with the leadership of the student groups and asked for their input about how we can better support them throughout their programs. They let us know that they needed to feel more centered and heard by our program faculty and they requested a faculty liaison – also a Person of Color – to be their point of contact with the program to be able to feel safer and more supportive in giving the program direct feedback. We also created a standing invitation for the student groups to address the CFT program during our quarterly community meetings.

4   Student Support

4.1   Recruitment and Retention of BIPOC Students

Faculty engaged in discussions on how to incorporate more inclusivity practices throughout our program, beginning with the admissions process. One of the pieces of feedback that had been outlined in the BSU letter was a complaint by one of our Black students about the admissions process to our program and the utilization of what they had perceived to be oppressive practices.

The practice they were referring to was a recent shift to us using video clips as points of discussion during our group interview process. We had previously used written case vignettes to facilitate group discussion during the prospective student interviews and had recently decided as a faculty that we wanted to create a more experiential activity as the prompt for discussion in the program. Additionally, we wanted to explicitly infuse both diversity in representation of the case vignette and conversations about racial injustice and white fragility into the interview experience.

In an effort to achieve this, we assembled a faculty work group made up of some of our Faculty Members of Color to develop this project. The final curated product was a series of clips from a feature film in which racial dynamics, power, privilege, and injustice are highlighted. In the interview activity, students are presented with five video clips from the film; each clip is then followed by a discussion question. The questions included prompts asking students to discuss personal reactions, attunement to power and privilege dynamics, as well as systemic reflection of a family system. The aim of this activity was to encourage prospective students to express themselves naturally and allow interviewers to review each prospective student against the values and qualities that the program desires in a student, which include values of anti-racism, inclusion, and self-awareness.

After initial implementation, we received feedback from the Counselors of Color student (CCS) support group that a Black student who participated in the interview process said that viewing the clips during the interview process felt unsafe as it mirrored personal experience to her. Additionally, it came across as if the process was developed by white faculty for white students; this made sense to us, as oftentimes the facilitators of the interview groups were white faculty members.

Of course this was not our intention in creating this interview protocol – far from it! But we realized that the process that we implemented left room for this to be experienced this way. In response, we made the decision to produce a more nuanced, edited video, which included an introduction given by a group of faculty members of color sharing with the interview group the objective of this portion of the interview (to bring challenging topics to the table for experiential discussion) along with a short explanation of the development of this process (faculty groups had worked in consultation with faculty of color to select the clips and develop the discussion questions) along with a brief content announcement before each clip was played (important because some of the clips included gun violence). Following the video clip, the discussion prompt was read by the same faculty members of Color on screen, rather than having the faculty members in the room read the questions, in an effort to provide continuity in the facilitation of the process, grounding it clearly in mission and purpose. We brought these changes back to the student group that had raised the concerns for their input, received their approval, and implemented the updates the following quarter.

5   Curriculum and Program Requirements

Our faculty work groups took time to reflect on our program's structure from top to bottom, including the academic schedules, use of course sequencing and tracks, and of course our curricula, in an effort to create an emotionally safer community in classrooms and in our department.

5.1   *Curriculum Review*

We reviewed all course syllabi and curricula to ensure that requirements include infusions of social justice through readings, class activities, and assignments. We decided to require that at least one course objective directly addresses intercultural competencies, inclusion, and racial awareness relevant to the course material, and that this needed to be stated clearly in the course syllabus. Here is an example of how this section looks in a syllabus for one of our Internship Case Consultation courses:

Anti-racism Objectives

- *How anti-racism and anti-oppression will be addressed in this course:* discourse through inclusion in course assignments and discussion about subjects of racism and oppression and their intersection with clinical work at internship sites.
- *Topics/content that will be discussed:* Some examples of the direct content of reflection incorporated into student assignments are:

Capstone Project Reflection: Perspectives on Multiculturalism and Social Justice (e.g., How do you integrate social justice, multicultural responsiveness, and anti-racism and anti-oppression frameworks into your clinical work? What is the role of the therapist in addressing oppression as it occurs indirectly or directly in your clinical work? In your community?)
Case Conceptualization sections on power and privilege reflections.

- *Anti-racism objectives for the course:* Reflect on and incorporate social justice, anti-oppression, and anti-racism frameworks into clinical work.
- *Readings/materials/resources used:*

McDowell, T., Knudson-Martin, C., & Bermudez, J.M. (2017). *Socioculturally Attuned Family Therapy*. Routledge. ISBN: 978-1138678217.

5.2   Teaching Anti-oppressive and Multicultural Curricula

A foundational course in our curriculum, "Multicultural Perspectives," also received a significant overhaul. This course has traditionally focused on cultural identification and acculturation, different worldviews, and their impact on therapeutic relationships. Desired outcomes included a student's vigilance regarding cultural differences, basic knowledge of minority groups, and a sense of cultural humility and curiosity. In recent years, however, Bergkamp et al. (2020) described a shift in the approach to teaching these courses, stating that the following:
The past decade has brought additional calls to extend the encatchment of these courses to address social justice, including issues of power, privilege, and oppression. This move is distinct, in so far as it begins to call into explicit focus the way in which cultural and identity differences have been historically co-opted into a contemporary and pervasive system of resource allotment. This moves cultural differences to power differences. It names issues of racism, sexism, and other major forms of oppression. It acknowledges the legacy of historic colonization and the ever-present colonial mentality...It gets political... It brings issues of power and privilege into the classroom...And, if done well, it gets messy. (p. 1).
While teaching courses that deal with privilege, oppression, and positionality is challenging for all faculty members, the burden is even greater for BIPOC faculty because the content in those courses require constant engagement with racial tension as BIPOC faculty strive to engage their students in discussion of the faculty's own lived experience (Anthym & Tuitt, 2019).
To address this, the faculty of color on our campus began by submitting a proposal to the university administration requesting that multicultural courses be co-taught by a BIPOC faculty member with another faculty member in order to off-set the burden. This approach is supported in the literature, finding that co-instruction requires that faculty foster collaborative working relationships and honor the need for inclusion and diversity (Lock et al., 2016) and encourages greater student reflection and awareness of their own learning process (Harter & Jacobi, 2018).

This approach helped faculty members feel supported in many ways. It allowed students the opportunity to learn from BIPOC faculty members while not placing all of the emotional labor for challenging conversations with the students about race solely on the BIPOC faculty. It also served to support non-BIPOC faculty members in having to navigate the challenges of leading racial conversations from the place of privilege as a white person.

5.3   Supervision and Internship

We realized that we also wanted to ensure opportunities for all of our students to learn from BIPOC faculty members throughout their program, and specifically in supervision during their internship. While previously we had one on-campus supervisor follow a group of students through their entire internship in their on-campus supervision group, we decided to make a shift to have two faculty members split a section over the course of the year (i.e., two quarters each), requiring that at least one of them identify as a BIPOC faculty member. This way, we could support centering BIPOC voices in the area of supervision for our students with 100% of our graduating students having received supervision from a BIPOC Program Clinical Supervisor for a substantial portion of their internship process.

Additionally, it was important to me that our internship program did not perpetuate for-profit businesses in affluent communities, but instead engaged our students in providing services to those who would otherwise go unserved or underserved. In recent years with the rise of private and group practices being approved for internship sites, we were seeing interns charge a relatively high rate for their services, unlike agency settings that accept state insurance. I began to grow concerned that practice owners (who by and large were white therapists in positions of financial privilege) were making "free money" off of intern labor, all the while still failing to serve clients who are in need of affordable mental health services. In return, we evaluated our internship process so that the program's social justice mission was directly tied to internship requirements and guidelines. We worked on revising the requirements for internship sites to affiliate with our program, including adding the requirement that the site must demonstrate that our interns were providing services for underserved populations. This process was implemented for all new sites, and still remains to be applied retroactively for existing sites.

5.4   Course Resources

Only 37% of the students surveyed indicated that faculty frequently included diverse, non-Eurocentric focused material and resources in every course; 12% indicated that diverse material was "never included" (Black Student Union, 2020). Faculty members were given the directive to make every attempt to reduce the

Eurocentric focus of course materials by including a balanced frequency of authors, academics, therapists, activists, and artists of Color. Any information that is utilized in a course should be sourced with appropriate attribution to authors, academics, therapists, activists, and artists.

We also recognized that an outcome of institutional racism in academia is that White academics and researchers are disproportionately represented in the literature. So as to accommodate for this imbalance we encouraged instructors to expand their use of course resources to include non-peer-reviewed articles, including books, videos, art exhibits, podcasts, music, and class activities that are created and developed by individuals of Color.

5.5 Student Engagement in Justice Activities

We created a program requirement of "social justice volunteer hours" that students must complete by the time they begin internship. This element was added based on feedback from faculty and students that more focused learning opportunities to practice social justice work were desired. We have also been working on creating student engagement opportunities, such as online networking times and workshops. While the pandemic has certainly slowed progress in these areas, future plans include hosting quarterly volunteer opportunities for students and faculty members to connect together around volunteer experiences.

6 Change at the Institutional Level

One of the major changes at the institutional level was a shift in the organization of our campus-wide faculty leadership team in 2020. Following an ongoing pattern of harmful experiences and interactions during all-faculty meetings, the BIPOC faculty on campus made the decision to boycott the meetings until white faculty members made a direct effort to address how institutional racism shows up at the university.

After months of back and forth, a new Faculty Leadership Team was formed to include a multiracial group of faculty members, all of whom cared deeply and felt committed to the mission to do anti-racism work as a collaborative. The goal of our new group was to work to promote repair and learning and a fundamental shift in the culture at the university – one that was aimed at developing an accountability process that would support BIPOC stakeholders in addressing racism in a way that is safe, without retaliation and rooted in restorative justice practices.

The group redesigned the structure of campus-wide faculty meetings to work toward an equitable and inclusive shared governance structure. We streamlined business meetings through the use of a consent agenda; this was helpful toward productivity and protecting faculty members of Color from harm, as previously, discussion around innocuous topics, like committee appointments, would regularly devolve into discussions laden with micro- and macro-aggressions toward faculty of color and other communities.

After much back and forth with university administration, we were able to coordinate the hire of an outside consultant to help facilitate conversations on developing an anti-racist framework for the university that will address the needs of all stakeholders, prioritizing BIPOC stakeholder needs and desires first. Through this, administration, faculty, staff, and students engaged in anti-racism and horizontal oppression work through monthly trainings, workshops, and caucus spaces.

In conjunction with these trainings, we required faculty attendance and participation, and included an addition of race-based caucus groups to create separate spaces for processing and learning around challenging racism personally and in the workplace. This work proved to be the most challenging. While these efforts were successful in some ways – for instance, BIPOC faculty members were shielded from having to witness white faculty members doing their own anti-racism work and processing by separating into race-based caucus groups – they were problematic in others. Despite the university operating from a social justice-oriented mission, it turns out that mandating faculty members to do anti-racism work was not well received by all and, for BIPOC faculty members, having to witness colleagues vocalize direct opposition to doing this work made for heightened tensions and fractured relationships between faculty members. Faculty members fought, outright refused to do the work and attend the meetings, and some even quit. I have never experienced anything quite like the heartbreak I felt when watching some of my closest and most trusted (white) colleagues refuse to vote to support taking action toward making our work spaces safer for BIPOC faculty, and then when the vote passed, turn in their resignations stating that their "values and mission no longer align with the direction the university and program are heading."

Perhaps I should not have been surprised. This experience is supported by research. Wise and Case (2013) described common obstacles to the experience of developing privilege awareness including defensiveness, judgment, guilt, shame, the myth of meritocracy, the learner's tendency to focus on marginalized identities, entitlement, fear of loss, and hopelessness in the face of injustice. These learner reactions are commonly attributed to those in leadership positions, especially BIPOC individuals.

7   Conclusion

To me, sometimes it felt like our faculty experience was simply an experiment for validating findings like I described in the preceding text. While I personally experienced enormous support by most of my colleagues within the program, the emotional wear of the entire multi-year process wore everyone down, and as the program leader, I felt the emotional brunt of it. Faculty morale showed a steady decline as more time passed, and as the point person for managing faculty concerns, it quickly took its toll on me. Even still, although I can sense we are on the road to healing and recovery, many of us are certainly worse for wear. I see it across my close faculty colleagues, those in other institutions, and most personally, in myself.

I feel grateful to be a part of a team of colleagues who have committed to doing the work of our mission, as I know that not all CFT faculties across the country are as open to this. Our program made choices to ensure that the voices of BIPOC authors, academics, and activists were well-represented in our course work. We evaluated our learning objectives and made decisions about how we could more actively engage ourselves as educators and our students as learners in social activism, moving beyond multicultural "lip service" in the classroom into active justice and service in our community. And yet, while I feel proud of the efforts our program has made to create safer, braver spaces for our BIPOC students, faculty, and staff, it has come with costs. BIPOC faculty members are *burned out*. The emotional burden has been great, and I often fear it is too much to bear. These battles have changed us.

I know I am not alone in this feeling. Research has found that BIPOC faculty routinely face subtle forms of discrimination and racism perpetrated by their colleagues, students, and institutions, to which they must respond with professionalism and poise (Kardia & Wright, 2004). These changes and efforts need to happen, and putting in this effort is *flat-out* hard. This journey has been taxing, vulnerable, infuriating, heartbreaking, and at the same time necessary. There is clearly so much work to still be done, and even on the worst days, I hold out hope that putting systems theory into practice will win out in the end, and a little bit of change at a time can go a long way in the end.

The question lingers for me: is it possible for our programs to sustain these changes and relationships at the same time? This duality sometimes feels impossible – other times, hopeful. In the meantime, we lean on each other. We hold space – both formally in meetings and informally through texts and personal check-ins – and we lean on the relationships that we have with one another. By doing this, I have found that each of us as individuals has the freedom to step in and out of spaces for advocacy, growth, introspection, frustration and anger, and rest and recovery, while continuing to move forward as a team and as a program. By keeping an eye on and tending to both the larger goals for the program as well as the individuals who make up our system, it seems we have the best shot at making change and doing so in the most sustainable way.

References

Anthym, M., & Tuitt, F. (2019). When the levees break: The cost of vicarious trauma, microaggressions and emotional labor for black administrators and faculty engaging in race work at traditionally white institutions. *International Journal of Qualitative Studies in Education, 32*(9), 1072–1093. https://doi.org/10.1080/09518398.2019.1645907

Bergkamp, J., Tudhope-Locklear, L., Fulmer, T., & Scheiderer, C. (2020). *BIPOC faculty burden and supports*. Unpublished manuscript. Clinical Psychology Department, Antioch University Seattle.

Black Student Union. (2020, July 9). *Hear our voices, letter to university provost on Black student experience*, Antioch University Seattle.

Harter, A., & Jacobi, L. (2018). "Experimenting with our education" or enhancing it? Co teaching from the perspective of students. I.E. *Inquiry in Education, 10*(2), 1–16.

Hayes, C., & Juárez, B. G. (2009). You showed your whiteness: You don't get a good white people medal. *International Journal of Qualitative Studies in Education, 22*(6), 729–744.

Kardia, D. B., & Wright, M. C. (2004). *Instructor identity: The impact of gender and race on* (p. 19). Faculty Experiences of Teaching. Center for Research and Learning on Teaching.

Lock, L., Clancy, T., Lisella, R., Rosenau, P., Ferreira, C., & Rainsbury, J. (2016). The lived experiences of instructors co-teaching in higher education. *Brock Education Journal, 26*(1), 22–35.

Solórzano, D. G., Ceja, M., & Yosso, T. J. (2000). Critical race theory, racial microaggressions, and campus racial climate: The experiences of African American college students. *Journal of Negro Education, 69*, 60–73.

Stotzer, R. L., & Hossellman, E. (2012). Hate crimes on campus: Racial/ethnic diversity and campus safety. *Journal of Interpersonal Violence, 27*(4), 644–661. https://doi-org.antioch.idm.oclc.org/10.1177/0886260511423249

Turner, C. S. V. (2002). Women of color in academe: Living with multiple marginality. *Journal of Higher Education, 73*, 74–93.

Wise, T., & Case, K. (2013). Pedagogy for the privileged: Addressing inequality and injustice without shame or blame. In *Deconstructing privilege: Teaching and learning as allies in the classroom*. Routledge Press.

Using Non-clinical Readings to Promote Cultural Attunement

Martha L. Morgan Gobert

My graduate studies in marriage and family therapy (MFT) left me feeling as though I did not quite belong. The models we studied were based on white middle-class people, which did not reflect my experiences as a Black woman. Often, I wondered how therapy works for Black people and other communities of color. These thoughts remained with me throughout my doctoral studies and as I entered academia as a professor. Educating marriage and family therapy students is part of my life's work and purpose, and I did not want my future students of color to experience the same feelings of disconnection I did.

In my master's degree program, we were introduced to the various family therapy models using Nichols and Schwartz's (2004) *Family Therapy Concepts and Methods*. Solution Focused Brief Therapy intrigued me, but I was not sure the model captured how I wanted to serve clients. In addition, I wanted to learn more about Satir's ideas, but there was no chapter dedicated to her work, and some in the field did not consider her work to be a true therapeutic model. I was drawn to Satir's work because she was the only female theorist in a field dominated by men. Over the course of my doctoral work, I was able to dive deeper into Satir's model and finally found my theoretical home. Like Satir, I had once wanted to become a teacher before eventually finding my way to the helping professions. Her curiosity and willingness to get to know people on a level that I had not seen in any other MFT model I had studied impressed me. She seemed warm and genuine, and I felt connected. The other theorists seemed distant, as if they were above me. Trying to fit myself into a white male therapist's role did not work. Now it makes sense since I am well past the point of trying to fit into a role that does not work for me. While becoming a therapist, however, I did not know how to be me and a therapist; I was

M. L. Morgan Gobert (✉)
UMass Global, Irvine, CA, USA
e-mail: martha.morgan@umassglobal.edu

© American Family Therapy Academy (AFTA) 2023
L. A. Nice, C. Eppler (eds.), *Social Justice and Systemic Family Therapy Training*,
AFTA SpringerBriefs in Family Therapy, https://doi.org/10.1007/978-3-031-29930-8_7

not sure if the authentic me would be welcomed by the professional world I was attempting to enter. The lack of representation made me doubt I belonged in the MFT field.

When I was developing my clinical voice – a reflection of myself steeped in Satir's work – I studied my master's program's own model, which combined a structural and strategic approach to treatment. My experience with this model was both excellent and limiting, as it seemed to suggest that there was only one way to be a therapist. While I appreciated both the structural and strategic approaches, there were some aspects of both that I did not like. I struggled with what felt like a demanding or dominant position as a therapist. It was important to me that clients had a voice in the direction of their healing. Clients needed to know that they had exactly what they needed to heal, so my role was more of a support than that of an all-knowing director.

Through these experiences, I was inspired to provide students with the opportunity to cultivate therapeutic alliances that reflect the personhood of both clients and therapists. I drew from my pre-clinical training in Human Resources Management (BAA) and Adult Education (MEd), which emphasized the importance of an integrative or multidisciplinary approach to teaching and learning. To facilitate my students' curiosity, learning, and capacity to engage with their future clients, I began incorporating non-clinical nonfiction or literature, from outside of the field of family therapy, into my classroom (e.g., autobiographies, non-fiction works on cultural dynamics).

The use of non-clinical texts that centered Black, Indigenous, and People of Color (BIPOC) voices and emphasized cultural experiences was missing from my marriage and family therapy training, which focused on systemic therapy and practice without fully taking racism, equity, and inclusion into account. To promote cultural sensitivity, I require my students to read nonfiction texts about real life experiences and potential solutions. Learners encounter real world stories of living in inequitable spaces (Stevenson, 2014) and how to be an anti-racist (Kendi, 2019). Since family systems theory taught me to value a multitude of perspectives, it only makes sense that I should include a wide range of readings in my theory and practice classes. Mental health issues are not the only issues clients bring to us, they also bring educational concerns, employment concerns, and legal concerns. Though I appreciate and understand the ethical mandate to stay within my scope of practice, I cannot ignore the impact of these varying issues on the work that goes on in therapy. When I think of the history of family therapy, I am intrigued by the various disciplines that the founders represented – anthropology, medicine, social work, among others (Nichols & Schwartz, 2004). The multidisciplinary perspective influenced the way we work as family therapists today, but we may have lost sight of this perspective somewhere along the way. I see my integration of reading material from outside family therapy as a way to re-engage with our roots, our past.

Humans are also valuable simply because they exist (Satir, 1972). With this value guiding me, it is my personal responsibility to ensure that students I train approach treatment from a socially just perspective. I fully agree with Bryan Stevenson (2014) who emphasizes the importance of justice in all areas of life. Justice must be at the center of everything we do as systemic therapists. If it is not, I am unsure of what we hope to accomplish as liberation is at the core of our work with clients. Including non-clinical texts when training MFT students is important in developing clinicians with a socially just lens, because these texts connect the real-world experiences that clients bring into therapy and the clinical understanding that students are developing in training.

1 Examples of Non-clinical Texts That Promote Cultural Attunement

A non-exhaustive list of texts I use in clinical education to promote cultural attunement include Stevenson (2014), Tatum (2017), DiAngelo (2018), Steele (2010), Takaki (2018), and Kruse and Zelizer (2019). Through the work I highlight in the following text, my students and I have expanded our perspectives on becoming therapists. Additional readings are provided at the end of this chapter.

Beverly Tatum, B. D. (2017). *Why Are All of the Black Kids Sitting Together in the Cafeteria*, focuses on identity development. Tatum (2017) highlights how we are racially socialized in our families of origin, and she gives voice to the influence primary caregivers have on racial identity development of young people. One of my students who identifies as white found the information Tatum shared particularly poignant; so much so that this student shared what the reading meant to them after finishing it and reported passing the book on to a family member. Another student expressed a desire to pass the book on to their children so they could learn about the development of white identity at a young age and become allies. Additionally, this student expressed frustration with not having been taught about these topics prior to attending graduate school. They stated, "I was initially annoyed about having to read an additional text in a course already packed full of readings, but this material is important. Not only will it help me be a better therapist, it's helping me become a better person."

Just Mercy highlights Bryan Stevenson's (2014) work with men, women, and children on death row. Although Stevenson is an attorney, his method of engaging clients and advocating for their interests is an important skill for new therapists to learn and hopefully adopt. Stevenson (2014) tells the story of incarcerated people and their relatives: a group that is often forgotten in society. Many therapists work with those who are or have been incarcerated, or their families, but often do not receive training in this area. I wanted my students to complete their masters training with some knowledge of potential clients who have had contact with the criminal justice system.

Stevenson's text introduces students to challenges within the criminal justice system and details his family history and his journey to law school. Throughout his story, he offers a glimpse into the journey of a first generation, low-income student to higher education. Stevenson's life and the lives of his clients are case studies of how families influence systemic work. With each of the stories he shares, the reader can see the systemic impact on both the individual and the family. Stevenson's own history of racism and justice shed light on how Black people can be seen by the justice system through a singular viewpoint – as criminals (Stevenson, 2014). His treatment by judges, prison guards, and the local police illustrates the plight of Black men in America; even those with advanced degrees from Ivy League colleges are not always protected (Stevenson, 2014). I believe that this information is crucial to helping new clinicians recognize the systemic nature of racism in the United States. For new clinicians, Stevenson's example of getting close or proximate to those many see as untouchable is invaluable. He demonstrated how important it is to see, listen, and really get to know his clients. I emphasize to new therapists the importance of doing the necessary work to get to know, see, and understand clients so that clinicians can provide culturally attuned care.

The revised edition of *A Different Mirror: A History of Multicultural America* provides a perspective on America through the eyes of the diverse groups that make up this nation (Takaki, 2008). Clinical students may gain historical knowledge they may not have otherwise acquired such as hearing directly from Native Americans, Chinese Americans, African Americans about their lived experience in the United States. This text shifts from the Anglo historical perspective of the United States to a BIPOC historical perspective. I believe this shift in historical perspective is important to learning because it allows students to appreciate the difference in the story when the storyteller is the one on the receiving end of injustice. Like Stevenson (2014) this work provides stories and examples for training clinicians to deepen their understanding of the role of culture in the United States and in the lives of clients they will serve.

In Fault Lines: A History of the United States Since 1974, Kruse and Zelizer (2019) offer a historical perspective that clinicians in training should read to deconstruct their ideas of dominant cultural norms. It provides an expanded perspective on racial, gender, and class divisions and highlights the systemic nature of oppression. The text also emphasizes the importance of zooming out or exploring a broader perspective when attempting to understand information. Developing this skill is essential for students as they prepare to become clinicians. Students gain a better understanding of the past's role in all aspects of the clients' lives by reading historical accounts with present-day significance. Studying the past can assist in understanding the present and identifying entry points for change in the future. Systemic therapists may use these strategies to work with clients to achieve the changes they want.

2 Using Justice-Oriented Texts in Clinical Education

The first time I used the non-clinical text, *Just Mercy* (Stevenson, 2014), to promote cultural attunement was in a group therapy class. The text was included to support a learning objective: students will be able to demonstrate knowledge of working effectively with diverse populations and understand the ethical and legal implications of meeting in groups. In class, the students were required to read the text and engage in discussion of the book using the discussion guide that can be downloaded from the authors' website.

In addition to class discussions the students were required to complete a reflection paper. To adequately prepare for the reflection paper students were encouraged to take notes on things discussed in class including their own insights, questions, curiosities, frustrations, etc., with reading the text. The students were required to write a two to three page reflection. The reflection paper was described as a self-reflective and introspective assignment, not a book report. Students were invited to consider how they might use the information from the text in service to their future clients.

For a pre-practicum course I taught, I incorporated bibliotherapy in a couple of different ways. First, students read texts based on being in a "book club." Several texts were provided as books for the book club. Students self-selected the book of their choice. Next, all students were required to read Tatum (2017). The course learning objective that aligned with this assignment was: Students have the basic core competencies to display both interpersonal and professional competence within clinical activities, service, scholarship, as well as collaborate with colleagues to practice in a variety of settings and with diverse populations.

The books included in the book club discussion groups were: DiAngelo, R. (2018), *White Fragility: Why It's So Hard for White People to Talk About Racism*; Steele, C. M. (2010), *Whistling Vivaldi: And Other Cues to How Stereotypes Affect Us*; and Kruse, K. M., & Zellzer, J. E. (2019), *Fault Lines: A History of the United States Since 1974*. The assignment invited students to discuss the book the group selected highlighting their expectations, anxieties, and concerns/questions related to the material in the book. Students were also invited to discuss ways the material will impact their work with clients.

Why Are All the Black Kids Sitting Together in the Cafeteria was used in the required readings at several points in the semester. The students would include their insights, reflections, new knowledge learned, and implications for therapy in the weekly discussion time. An alternate format for incorporating these texts in a pre-practicum course was via a weekly podcast. The same text from the book club described previously was used as well as Tatum (2017). For this format students were placed into groups of three to four, and each group was assigned one of the books listed in the preceding text. Students were invited to set a time to meet with their group to record a video or audio podcast where they discuss the readings. Students could record their podcast with the format of choice.

To complete the podcast, students were asked to work collaboratively to develop an outline of the major conversation points/topics they planned to discuss. The conversation needed to focus on the students' reactions and responses to the assigned readings for the week. The key areas of focus for the discussion were on demonstrating they had read the material and reflected on the implications for their future work with clients. All students in the groups were expected to contribute to the conversation. The students rotated the moderator for each conversation and the conversations were approximately 50 minutes in length. The students needed to record the conversation and submit one recording for the group.

3   What Have Been the Outcomes of Bibliotherapy?

The inclusion of these texts has broadened students' perspectives, both personally and professionally. Students expressed frustration at not having been exposed to this information until graduate school. Several people shared how the new knowledge has affected their interactions with family and friends. As shared earlier, some have shared the books with family, others plan to use the books to teach their own children, and others shared having a deeper understanding of the challenges their minority family and friends experience.

After reading *Just Mercy*, my students and I have a debriefing discussion about their thoughts and the aspects of the text they will use during their future client contacts. In my experience, most students were initially annoyed and confused by my inclusion of the text. I have used this text several times, and the initial debriefing discussion always focuses on the students' lack of awareness surrounding the criminal justice system. They are often shocked to learn that children are held in adult prisons and tried as adults, and many are surprised by the way women and people with mental illness are treated. Future therapists need to recognize the negative effects of these types of imprisonment on the family. One student shared that she had found a new area of professional focus. The student, like Bryan Stevenson, wanted to dedicate their life to serving families involved in the criminal justice system. It is exciting to watch students transition from frustrated to curious to engaged to passionate based on their required reading.

I was surprised by the response of the students from minoritized backgrounds when I used DiAngelo's (2018) *White Fragility* as part of the texts for the book club. The students selected the book but were unhappy that I allowed them to select the text instead of requiring their white classmates to read it. When I asked why they felt this way, they responded, "it's for white people and the author is trying to help them understand their issues." My question to them was, "Did you learn anything that will help you better understand the response of your classmates, other white people you know, and white clients in your future practice?" The students said they did, but they felt that white students in the program needed the information more than they did. As someone who encourages people to make choices, I reminded the students they were free to make the choice in their book just like every other student in the class. However, the consequences of our choices are not always up to us, even though we have some agency in our choices. In our class discussion time, I encouraged the students to be very intentional about how they discussed the text while in class and as they created connections outside of the classroom.

4   Future Directions

At the time of this writing, I am teaching a course focused on human diversity to master's level mental health students. The course, designed by a colleague, had limited space for additional texts. I have incorporated videos of Bryan Stevenson discussing his work to expose students to material outside of the required reading. For example, one video focused on the development of the Legacy Museum and monument. Another video focused on the importance of hope and proximity. Although I was not able to assign the texts, I appreciate videos that relate to the content of the texts as those videos allowed my students to make connections to the material. I also include a book recommendation almost every week to encourage them to be independent learners.

In future classes, I plan to share portions of Martin Luther King Jr.'s (1963) "Letter from a Birmingham Jail" with the students to deepen their understanding of race and racism. I believe the content of this letter is relevant to the state of the world today and therefore will be useful. This letter written by Dr. King while in a Birmingham jail highlights his commitment to nonviolence and social justice. We will discuss Dr. King's role as an agitator after listening to portions of the letter, since it is often overlooked when discussing his work. We will also discuss how the information will help the students better serve their future clients, what they notice about the content of Dr. King's letter today, and how they see themselves advocating based on what they learn from Dr. King's letter. Through their answers to these questions, they will be able to consider where we have been, where we are headed, and what role they may play in shaping our future. I also hope that the reading will encourage them to gain a deeper understanding of Dr. King beyond the "I Have a Dream" speech.

Continually exposing students to knowledge beyond their field is my goal beyond this course. Since I am a systems thinker, I believe that understanding client needs should not be limited to marriage and family therapy. I believe that just as systems theory taught us to look beyond individuals to understand the problems clients bring to therapy, we also need to look beyond our field in order to understand the lived experience of the clients we get to serve.

References

DiAngelo. (2018). *White fragility: Why it's so hard for white people to talk about racism*. Beacon Press.

Kendi, I. X. (2019). *How to be an antiracist*. Random House.

King, M. L., Jr. (1963). *Letter from a Birmingham jail*. Penguin Classics.

Kruse, K. M., & Zelizer, J. E. (2019). *Fault lines: A history of the United States since 1974*. W.W. Norton & Company.

Nichols, M. P., & Schwartz, R. C. (2004). *Family therapy: Concepts and methods* (6th ed.). Pearson.

Satir, V. (1972). *Peoplemaking*. Science and Behavior Books, Inc.

Steele, C. M. (2010). *Whistling Vivaldi: And other cues to how stereotypes affect us*. W. W. Norton and Company.

Stevenson, B. (2014). *Just mercy: A story of justice and redemption*. Speigel & Grau.

Takaki, R. (2018). *A different mirror: A history of multicultural America*. Back Bay Books.

Tatum, B. D. (2017). *Why are all the black kids sitting together in the cafeteria? And other conversations about race* (2nd ed.). Basic Books.

Decolonizing Higher Education Through Incorporating Antiracist Pedagogy in Doctoral Students' Academics, Mentorship, and Training

Branson Boykins and Sarah K. Samman

1 Multiculturally Focused Training Programs

A goal of any multiculturally focused training program is to meet the needs of a racially and culturally diverse student body. In our view, training programs in name only, without actionable commitment to antiracist pedagogy, are inherently problematic and lack opportunities for growth. In this chapter, we briefly discuss the importance of antiracist positioning as well as introduce ourselves and our social contexts to punctuate how our experiences inspired us to commit to multicultural and antiracist pedagogy. We share the ways we learned from our experiences, including combating our own assumptions and passivity toward an evolving multicultural and antiracist academic journey.

Dr. Ibram Kendi's (2019) controversial publication *How to Be an Antiracist* could not have come at a better time as we worked through our own antiracist journeys, especially as it pertains to our work in academia. Everyone deserves to feel confident academically. We imagine a world without carrying the burden of internalized racist and prejudiced ideologies that convince people with lesser privilege that they are worth less. Accordingly, faculty called to ally ship must intentionally combat the stereotypes, prejudices, and biases that reinforce these ideas that are believed to be rooted within people. There cannot be neutrality in any academic program or experience when it promotes ideologies grounded in policies that hinder the right to academic confidence and success (Kendi, 2019). For this reason, it is critical for faculty to challenge inequity by supporting applicants and students of the global majority differently toward systemic equity and justice.

B. Boykins (✉) · S. K. Samman
Alliant International University, San Diego, CA, USA
e-mail: branson.boykins@alliant.edu

© American Family Therapy Academy (AFTA) 2023
L. A. Nice, C. Eppler (eds.), *Social Justice and Systemic Family Therapy Training*,
AFTA SpringerBriefs in Family Therapy, https://doi.org/10.1007/978-3-031-29930-8_8

To further understand our dedication to this positioning, we would like to briefly situate ourselves within the context of our commitment to antiracism. I (Branson) identify as a Black or African American (AA) cisgender, heterosexual man and an Associate Professor in the Couple and Family Therapy Program at Alliant International University in Irvine, CA. I am originally from Detroit, MI, and received my terminal doctorate in counseling psychology from Western Michigan University. My family originates from several parts of the United States (U.S.; e.g., Augusta, GA; Cleveland, OH, and Detroit, MI), and consists of highly educated professionals who value education, service, racial pride, and community. I have provided counseling services in a variety of settings (e.g., schools, university counseling centers, community mental health clinics, an incarceration center, and youth residential), many of which offered me opportunities to work with racial minorities, especially AAs. I owe a great deal of my training and education to a select group of AA mentors in my masters and doctoral programs and am fortunate to say that I had an all AA doctoral committee. These experiences furthered my passion to serve in academia and research while specializing in areas of multicultural psychology, AA psychology, men's issues, and contemporary forms of bias and discrimination.

Growing up, I experienced various forms of racial marginalization through micro- and macro-aggressions (Sue et al., 2019). White teachers lowered expectations, ignored my opinions, or said I was lucky to have made educational strides in the Detroit Public School System. Later on, my supervisors assumed that I would be able to work clinically with AAs despite receiving little to no training on this underserved population before my doctorate. As a professor, I continue to experience similar problems. Students have reported believing in the stereotypic images of Black men as angry and aggressive versus smooth or Black Cool Pose. They shared expectations that I would match these images and have written overtly racist comments about me in my course evaluations, cursed at me during office hours and meetings, frequently argued against established research on racial bias, and even made comments regarding my attire such as "being dressed as a cute boy." Withstanding these constant reminders of institutional racism within academia has taught me valuable lessons regarding student mentorship, academia, racial battle fatigue, picking battles, feeling unheard, forced compliance, and knowing my worth.

I (Sarah) worked as adjunct faculty for two years prior to joining Alliant International University in San Diego, California, and am now in my sixth year and an Associate Professor in the Couple and Family Therapy Program. I identify as a White cisgender, heterosexual, bicultural (Middle Eastern and European American), binational (Saudi and United States citizen), bilingual (Arabic and English), and religious and spiritual Muslim woman. I live in a larger, predominantly able body, am middle class, formally educated, and am a wife, mother, intersectional feminist, therapist, and professor navigating the complexities of academia. My immediate and extended family system values the building of knowledge, skill sets, and expertise as well as passion for their chosen careers. This directly influenced my desire to excel in the field of marriage and family therapy (MFT) and I began my journey providing therapy services in inpatient and outpatient addiction and rehabilitation services, behavioral health clinics, as well as a transplant institute. I earned my terminal doctoral degree in Marital and Family Therapy from Loma Linda University in California.

I have personally experienced marginalization because of my intersecting identities due to patriarchal, political, and religious motives. Interestingly, I am often described as a Person of Color (POC) for presenting as an overtly practicing, but still White, Muslim woman. I have been explicitly asked how I could possibly call myself "an intersectional feminist and be a Muslim at the same time." I have had a few male students challenge me during office hours and tell me I should be "submissive" like I am expected to be in my "home country," implying not only a prejudicial belief, but one that excludes me from considering the U.S. my home. I have been explicitly described as a "foreigner" who does not understand "American culture" due to my paternal lineage and despite my complex sociopolitical maternal history in Northern America. This includes identifying as one of the First Families of Virginia and acknowledging the lineage of ancestors that enslaved Black individuals and families in the South.

2   Diverse Family Therapy Programs: Our Antiracist Vision

We learned quickly that choosing careers in academia would require commitment to actively intervene in power processes undermining diversity, equity, and inclusion. There were times when we felt powerless in the face of larger and more influential institutions, where the promotion of diversity and antiracist pedagogy would challenge the white majority perspective, and we might be considered nuisances or agitators. We knew that promoting a truly multiculturally focused training program would require that the institution as a whole – in addition to both core and adjunct faculty – take action. Steps toward this include faculty demonstrating awareness of their own social locations, then highlighting key components and interventions in their course content and the overall academic experience that reinforces racial inequality. This requires a keen awareness of the steep learning curve required to delicately balance the power dynamics involved.

3   Representation Does Matter: Commitment to a Diverse Faculty and Student Body

One of the ways we committed to an antiracist lens is by acknowledging the power that privileged communities have to describe, categorize, and treat others based on race, from historically describing Black and Brown folks as colored, to labeling them as minorities, to adopting the more person centered term in POC. We have first-hand knowledge of the ways Individuals of the Global Majority (IGM) commonly experience disparities in treatment in predominantly White communities

(Kendi, 2019). These are further exacerbated by disparities by White passing or White adjacent individuals from their own communities. We acknowledge that categorization has been an integral part of reducing individuals and communities to often superficial and decontextualized features. This is exceedingly problematic as 80% of the world's nearly eight billion inhabitants are considered POC (Campbell-Stephens, 2020). Thus, part of our antiracist approach is to actively deemphasize White centered and exclusionary terminology to be more accurate and inclusive.

4 Diverse Faculty and Students: Leaning into and Utilizing Our Intersecting Identities

When searching for our professional academic home, we applied to institutions that focused on building multiculturally diverse training programs that have racially and culturally diverse faculty, higher administration, and staff. Diverse faculty composition is critical for many reasons, including learning from unfortunate experiences with and commitment to combating marginalizing and discriminatory processes in academia. Part of our approach as early career educators was to be honest about the strengths of our program and the ways it may be lacking and where it could benefit from additional attention. We were also aware of the importance of acknowledging and understanding our static as well as dynamic social locations and intersecting identities as we navigate these processes. We learned that growth toward antiracist work generally evolves from a diverse faculty composition that then encourages and admits a diverse student cohort.

4.1 Diverse Applicants: Equitable Admissions Processes

One of the ways we committed ourselves to more equitable admissions processes is by doing away with requiring the Graduate Record Examination (GRE) scores or the strict adherence to a minimum grade point average (GPA). We decided to take an active approach to the process and acknowledge that a large majority of IGM, especially women, report that they lack the knowledge (i.e., mentorship, research skills) and abilities (i.e., financial resources, test taking scores) to navigate the application process for college in general, and postgraduate education in particular. Even though the technical aspects of the admissions process are beyond the scope of faculty responsibilities, we have taken steps to ensure we do not refuse applicants who do not meet all of the program's predetermined admissions criteria, that is, official transcripts with GPA, prerequisites, letters of recommendation, essay reflecting the fit for the program and research interests, curriculum vitae, etc.

I (Sarah) and my colleagues at the San Diego Branch recommend scheduling individual interviews with two faculty members if students do not appear to meet all the predetermined criteria for an interview. This provides applicants with the opportunity to express any concerns they may have regarding their application and fit for the program. We request examples of how the student has learned a skill set or has a plan to achieve success in the program and in the field in general. Additionally, we learned the value of developing a list of multiculturally informed admissions interview questions, as shown in Table 1, that encourage IGM to highlight their academic and interpersonal strengths and potential.

4.2 Diverse Classroom Experiences

Discussions in the classroom and experiential activities that elicit dialogue from multiple perspectives have been some of the biggest rewards of implementing antiracist practices. As a student, I (Branson) recall several instances where I attended a Predominantly White Institution (PWI) and felt isolated as the only Black male in the classroom. I often felt pressured to "represent" all Black students or Black men when topics arose that connected to my Black identity. These types of experiences were psychologically harmful and impacted my academic performance and sense of belonging and comfort within the learning environment. Encouraging a diverse student body challenges the pressure faced by students of the global majority to be a voice for their community when interacting with individuals with more privilege such as White, White passing, or White adjacent faculty or peers.

Table 1 Multiculturally informed admissions interview questions

1. What draws you as an applicant to this profession/program?
2. What personal/diversity strengths would you bring to your academic journey as well as therapy room?
3. What personal/diversity weaknesses or biases might you bring to your academic journey as well as therapy room?
4. Tell us something about yourself, community, or interests that we would not get from your application materials?
5. What drew you to the field/profession and what challenges might you have overcome to get here?
6. What are the populations with which you resonate, have a passion for, or with whom you work well?
7. What are the populations with which you have historically struggled or anticipate you may experience difficulties?
8. What skills have you developed to manage potential difficulties?
9. What is an example of a time when it was difficult or painful to hear some feedback, especially if diversity related, and what did you do with the feedback provided?
10. Where do you see yourself 5 years after graduation and why?

4.3 Blocking the Demand for Emotional Labor

Another common challenge to antiracist learning spaces is determining whether or not we should address microaggressions publicly or privately. When addressing them in a public space, we have found it helpful to mindfully and respectfully challenge the student's request for emotional labor and redirect attention away from the IGM. We can challenge privilege in those moments by reflecting, "Those are some great thoughts and there might be areas of growth that some of you might benefit from. What is important is to ask ourselves what is the purpose of the question? If it seems out of curiosity, what are the potential areas of growth? What are some biases we might have held and how might we do better knowing what we know now? What are some biases that we still hold and how can we dismantle them? I can help point you to some authors who've put in the emotional labor to address questions like these."

4.4 Making Space and Challenging Invisible Privilege

At times, students feel compelled to express feelings of guilt or shame about not having to "deal with" racial issues. I (Sarah) personally fell into that shameful feeling as a White woman, speaking to how I could simply take off my headscarf and benefit from my Whiteness. However, I quickly realized that I was occupying space that was not mine. My failure to stay in my lane unintentionally silenced important voices. While painful and embarrassing when redirected to focus on the experiences of my peers from the global majority, it was necessary. Managing student reactions such as defensiveness and blame is also important. As faculty, I try to validate as well as join in the discomfort and normalize the reaction. I let them know that I understand it might be hard to acknowledge the more powerful parts of the self when we have a tendency to attune to the less powerful and more victimized experiences of ourselves. When we know better, we can do better.

4.5 Mentorship as an Intentional Diversity-Centered Process

In both our past experiences as students and current experiences as faculty, we have found that students experiencing marginalization often have intersecting identities that present as additional barriers for our consideration. For example, they may identify as first- or second-generation immigrants or international students struggling with language barriers, first-generation college, graduate, or doctoral students, or students experiencing financial burdens or hardships. We have heard their fears of being "found out" and proven inadequate, worrying about faculty disappointment, and feeling burdensome. As faculty, we need to be intentionally mindful of how each student's various intersecting identities can impact their learning style, interpersonal relationships with faculty and peers, reactions to learned materials, and potential and challenging barriers to their success.

Based on our personal and anecdotal experiences, we have found that students may avoid seeking out mentorship for the preceding reasons. Because of this, we ensure we briefly and openly speak about how our identities intersect within and outside of academia as well as create space for dialogue for students from marginalized communities in the classroom. More specifically, having personally (Branson) attended PWIs, but still benefited from AA faculty mentorship, I have learned to take the responsibility to give back to future generations. Through a variety of approaches. I provide real world examples of the encouragement and hardships I faced as a student and as a beginning therapist so they feel validated in their experiences and hopeful about the future.

We also speak to our confidence as faculty in our decision to accept our students and invest in their success. We make a point of speaking to how comparisons among peers undermine each of their individual and contextual goals and could result in internalized shame. Shame is a powerful antagonist that leads to further isolation and blocks desire to connect with others. So it makes sense that we normalize confusion, stress, and overwhelm in an effort to level the playing field and promote self- and other-compassion and grace. We try to serve as role models and offer encouragement and reassure students that we all have areas of potential and growth. We encourage them to actively audit their skill sets and develop confidence in their ability to learn and succeed just as competently as any other student within the program.

When considering students' fear of inadequacy, we work to provide space for conversations about career development and professionalism for those who may be unaware of ways to make the most of their mentorship experiences. Examples may include discussing differences between a résumé and curriculum vitae, the importance of a cover letter and what it should include and why, the benefits of networking, especially when attending conferences and symposia, how to research and apply for fellowships and scholarships, and how to be involved in leadership positions in university-related organizations. All of this is critical for the development of a strong, culturally diverse cohort, where students who were originally perceived as "weak" applicants are viewed as just as strong as their peers by the end of their academic training.

Lastly, it is helpful to keep a log of which students could benefit from additional mentorship, particularly those who appear reluctant to seek guidance. We make note of our observations during faculty meetings to set these students up for success in their relationships with other faculty and staff. Part of our goal for student mentorship is to remind students of the possibility of succeeding at the highest levels, even when reporting suffering from "imposter syndrome." This syndrome is often used as an explanation of internal struggles that one has to overcome with toxic positivity such as "just be confident," "ignore your self-doubts," or "don't wait until you're offered a seat at the table." However, in reality, this phenomenon is deeply contextual and reflects a power imbalance in which those in power decide what is valued and sought out and exclude the multiple and equally valid skill sets that marginalized populations and communities can and should be able to offer toward a globally rich and meaningful experience.

4.6   Challenges Implementing Antiracist Pedagogy

Serving as a multiculturally informed and antiracist faculty member has presented challenges, both personally and professionally. Among these challenges are the asymmetry between multicultural/diversity course intent and outcome, as well as challenging student–faculty interactions, including those requiring additional faculty labor and further emotional burden.

4.7   Asymmetry Between Course Intent and Outcome

Graduate training programs may strive to incorporate a multiculturally infused training program where clinical and developmental theories are contextually viewed through lenses of diversity, inclusion, power, privilege, and racism. However, training programs seem to be falling short of this ideal vision when superficially discussing topics of bias, discrimination, and racism and in ways that reinforce the status quo (Beitin et al., 2008; Yzaguirre et al., 2022). We therefore ask our readers, if in such a program, how might you assess if you are accomplishing your goal? How might you intentionally encourage the absorption of legitimate and valuable emic experiences of diversity? How might you avoid maintaining institutional racism when accepting and disseminating only the work of white men or even white feminists?

4.8   Acknowledging Faculty-Related Challenges and Biases

Teaching a multicultural or diversity informed course is challenging and we certainly experienced a variety of feelings, pressures, and unease due to multiple stressors in combination with our intersecting identities. Challenges we have faced as early career faculty included how best to educate students, how much attention we pay to specific racial or cultural groups, self of the teacher and therapist exploration, education about power, privilege, and microaggressions, and integrating cross-cultural interventions within systemic theories. We have also learned that we must explore our own biases and potential for them to infuse the learning experience.

I (Sarah) have insecurities as a White woman teaching diversity courses. I have learned that no matter how much I prepare in advance, each classroom or system will introduce opportunities for conflict, yet also have opportunities for resolution.

I have found that self-compassion and self-grace are critical. I continue to remind myself to move beyond the didactic, content-based parts of the discussion to a more relational, process-based approach to student discussion. Understanding that faculty do not have all the answers and often have their own biases relieves me of some pressure, and allows me to model how to address conflict and disagreements. It also allows me to demonstrate how to manage discussions when not all opinions have equal grounding, weight, or legitimacy.

4.9 Acknowledging Student-Related Challenges and Biases

When teaching diversity courses, I (Branson) identify several internal goals grounded in encouraging student self-growth and a better understanding of their identities as racial and cultural beings. I attempt to create spaces for challenging dialogues where students can express their worldviews, while also understanding how these views might differ from or minimize someone else's. This is why it is absolutely critical that we avoid tone policing marginalized voices in order to soften the real struggles of racism and make them more palatable to those with more privilege. For example, a few students of privilege reported that they or their families believe racism no longer exists, any reports are exaggerated, and IGM use it as a "race card" to advance academically or professionally. Though difficult conversations to navigate, we are grateful for opportunities to invite disagreement and to see student comfort in expressing views that might be contradictory to others. I (Branson) attempt to listen to the students' perspectives while also providing various sources of information (e.g., personal testimonials, self-disclosure, research articles, and current socio-political events) to highlight the pervasiveness of the belief as well as limitations of their argument and how it may likely influence interpersonal relationships and clinical interactions.

4.10 Challenging Student–Faculty Interactions and Relationships

As is expected, we have experienced microaggressions, racial battle fatigue, compassion fatigue, and burnout from covert as well as overt negative and harmful course experiences (Bradley, 2005; Bradley & Holcomb-McCoy, 2004; Salazar, 2009). As alluded to in previous sections, a key, but emotionally laborious, skill when teaching antiracist and multiculturally focused coursework is developing negotiation and gentle maneuvering skills. This is where faculty must prepare compelling arguments and persuasive points to help educate privileged students who reject concepts based on anecdotal evidence, particularly personal ones based on their own marginalized social locations. We have had our fair share of students who outright reject or minimize concepts such as White privilege, institutional racism, mental health disparities, or the need for cross-cultural interventions. We often validate and empathize with areas of underprivileged social location before challenging their privilege; for example, by highlighting that they may have experienced hardship due to financial hardships, but not due to the compounding effects of the color of their skin. Regardless of how well we may highlight relevant terminology, trends in research, personal experiences, client experiences, and historical foundations in a tactful and non-threatening way, faculty must prepare for dismissive responses such as "I guess we have to agree to disagree" as though they are equally valid positions.

Faculty and program directors should be aware of the likelihood of receiving criticism or negative feedback from students because they are tasked with challenging internal biases, promoting cultural and racial awareness and growth, and resistance to antiracist pedagogy. For example, we received numerous negative evaluations that were not connected to actual classroom content or instruction. Students have reported that we were "mean" and "intimidating" as well as fearful that I (Branson) was going to label them as "racist." It is understandable that students might use an evaluation to anonymously vent their frustrations; however, these often showcase their prejudicial biases toward us as the instructors, and these statements have lasting impacts on us.

We have been fortunate that they have fallen in the hands of supportive leadership and administrators rather than in the hands of those who reinforce a fear within us of losing our contracts, or use them against us when seeking promotion, salary increase, new employment, or tenure. And although there is a dilemma for faculty who have to weigh the cost of teaching antiracist pedagogy at the expense of their well-being, professional reputation, and future in academia, they may find it well worth the risk long term as we did. We believe that the active commitment to continued professional growth and the application of antiracist pedagogy is a worthy endeavor and one that results, at the very least, in the passive support and uplifting of marginalized students and their allies' academic and professional experiences.

5 Concluding Recommendations: Antiracist Action Items

First and foremost, faculty benefit greatly from acknowledging and challenging their racist and prejudicial ideals. Faculty and program leaders must practice acknowledging how their identity, values, and beliefs shape and inform the culture, mission, and vision of their respective training programs. Faculty should routinely engage in a life-long process of antiracist work beginning with looking inward and asking for personal and professional consultation regarding areas of growth during the endeavor. This type of introspective work can lay the foundation for program transformation and liberation.

Second, we recommend the clear commitment and advocacy for visibility and representation in any faculty and student body. Once a program adopts an antiracist training focus, department heads and faculty with institutional power have a responsibility to commit and maintain a diverse faculty and student cohort. Intentionality, as we have discussed, is key. Programs can audit which faculty take on an antiracist vision and how to recruit, support, and retain them. These programs can also actively adapt to equitable application processes and contextual support for these students once admitted. As Kendi (2019) described, for students and faculty of the global majority and/or represent marginalized identities, intentionally treating them differently by considering their actual rather than assumed resources will yield equitable opportunities and outcomes.

Third, programs benefit from the nuance of diversity-centered mentorship considerations. An antiracist training program should value mentorship and lean into how intersecting identities promote difficult and challenging discussions and experiences. Faculty must be mindful of the types of students who are likely to ask for help or feel confident in their ability, and those who may need additional support and guidance. Therefore, we call for intentionality in mentorship from a social justice and antiracist framework – one that creates affirming dialogue, support, and resources for all students including those who are likely to be left behind because of systemic oversight that often reinforces their fear of asking for help.

Fourth, we want to reiterate the obvious. Faculty self-care is critical to the success of antiracist work. Faculty such as ourselves are likely to experience challenges, burnout, and discriminatory encounters in the pursuit of an antiracist training program. We urge faculty to find avenues and support for self-care such as personal therapy, exercise, religious-spiritual support, as well as connecting with like-minded faculty within one's program, institution, or field.

We hope that through our stories and action items you also hear a call to personally reflect, consider, and suggest programmatic changes, and find the courage and dedication to challenge your training programs as they currently are. We hope you practice self- and other-compassion and recognize all the things you have done well and the areas in which you could benefit from continued growth. Perform an audit of your work and what values and direction you wish to lead in your training program, classroom, and own personal life. This work takes time, includes hurdles, and can be painful and exhausting. Yet we push through, and we hope you will join us and lend us your expertise as well.

References

Beitin, B., Duckett, R., & Fackina, P. (2008). Discussions of diversity in a classroom: A phenomenological study of students in an MFT training program. *Contemporary Family Therapy, 30*(4), 251–268. https://doi.org/10.1007/s10591-008-9072-4

Bradley, C. (2005). The career experiences of African American women faculty: Implications for counselor education programs. *College Student Journal, 39*(3), 518–528.

Bradley, C., & Holcomb-McCoy, C. (2004). African American counselor educators: Their experiences, challenges, and recommendations. *Counselor Education and Supervision, 43*(4), 258–273. https://doi.org/10.1002/j.1556-6978.2004.tb01851.x

Campbell-Stephens, R. (2020). *Global majority*. Unpublished paper affiliated with Leeds Becket University UK. https://www.leedsbeckett.ac.uk/-/media/files/schools/school-of-education/final-leeds-beckett-1102-global-majority.pdf

Kendi, I. X. (2019). *How to be an antiracist*. One World.

Salazar, C. F. (2009). Strategies to survive and thrive in academia: The collective voices of counseling faculty of color. *International Journal for the Advancement of Counseling, 31*(3), 181–198. https://doi.org/10.1007/s10447-009-9077-1

Sue, D. W., Alsaidi, S., Awad, M. N., Glaeser, E., Calle, C. Z., & Mendez, N. (2019). Disarming racial microaggressions: Microintervention strategies for targets, white allies, and bystanders. *American Psychologist, 74*(1), 128. https://doi.org/10.1037/amp0000296

Yzaguirre, M. M., PettyJohn, M. E., Tseng, C. F., Asiimwe, R., Fang, M., & Blow, A. J. (2022). Marriage and family therapy masters students' diversity course experiences. *Journal of Feminist Family Therapy: An International Forum, 34*(1–2), 15–37. https://doi.org/10.1080/08952833.2022.2052534

Person of the Therapist: An Ethical Training Model

Anthony Pennant and Zain Shamoon

This chapter calls for a paradigm shift in clinical graduate programs regarding their fundamental commitment to matters of anti-oppression and personal attunement to cultural dynamics in therapy. We review the Person of the Therapist (POTT; Aponte & Kissil, 2014) training based on our experiences for its utility in developing socio-culturally attuned and anti-oppressive therapists in the field of family therapy. This chapter begins with an introduction of the authors, as well as areas of conviction we hold given our experiences as professors, researchers, and clinicians thus far. In our estimation, self-work in family therapy training has filtered through an academic status quo that centers learning styles not meant for diverse populations. We will speak to our advocacy for a change in the culture, where family therapy training becomes more personal; an impetus we feel strongly about, given that the work of therapy is personal.

The Person of the Therapist model is a framework of clinical training developed by Harry Aponte (Aponte & Kissil, 2014), which transforms the historical understanding of countertransference in the therapeutic relationship, and invites clinicians to utilize a more comprehensive view of themselves, including their wounds, to create real experiences for the individual they are treating. We hope to champion this model in our effort to call for a necessary culture shift in our field, toward greater acceptance of therapist personhood and enhanced sociocultural attunement.

A. Pennant (✉) · Z. Shamoon
Antioch University, Seattle, CA, USA
e-mail: apennant@antioch.edu

© American Family Therapy Academy (AFTA) 2023
L. A. Nice, C. Eppler (eds.), *Social Justice and Systemic Family Therapy Training*,
AFTA SpringerBriefs in Family Therapy, https://doi.org/10.1007/978-3-031-29930-8_9

1   Person of the Therapist: Main Components

Clinicians can be trained in the POTT model in their master's program or in the post-graduate experience. The POTT model aims to incorporate a clinician's previous experiences in past relationships as a tool of connection and intervention, providing clients a genuine therapeutic encounter. The heart of the model is the understanding of how clinicians manage their relationships through distress. This is called a signature theme (Aponte & Kissil, 2014). Potential trainees are able to name and develop their signature themes through three phases of oversight and training. Those phases are: The Knowledge of Self, The Access of Self, and The Use of Self. The Knowledge of Self is the exploration of the person's signature theme. The Access of Self is the practice of identifying what may be happening in the here and now for a person in the midst (or absence) of a signature theme being triggered. Lastly, the Use of Self is the practice of utilizing the here and now experiences of the clinician for the good of the client. This may or may not look like self-disclosure, but the active *use* of the therapist as a tool/intervention is what is important.

2   Person of the Therapist: An Ethical Imperative

We take the position that clinicians in training deserve robust methods on the development of their *ethical* selves, including through mistakes they make; these are opportunities for self-reflection and growth according to the POTT-training model. Trainees move through the POTT model over three academic quarters, engaging with each of the three themes. In our view, these themes allow trainees to develop sociocultural and ethical attunement, by way of providing students experiential opportunities to understand where and when their biases occur and how that is ethically managed in clinical practice. For instance, our students are asked to consider how they might respond to moments where they have offended clients, including oppressive statements toward others' identities. Here, trainees are given a multitude of opportunities to critically think and respond to in the moment experiences, whether this be in a classroom setting or supervision.

In the first phase of the training, this is conducted through signature theme presentations, where trainees write-up their current understanding of their signature themes: the typical patterns by which people relate to close others, their professional work, and life overall. For example, my (ZS) signature theme has to do with desiring belonging and closeness, and I used to back away from this as a clinician for fear that that type of humanity was unethical.

In the second phase of the model (access of self), trainees are provided multiple opportunities to *access self:* scan for their sensory responses and physical awareness of self that provides a cue that something is happening. This is used as a consistent grounding technique, and trainees are encouraged to consider how sensory responses are related to the signature themes they reflected on in phase one. In addition, the art of accessing one's inner self (and reactions) can provide greater understanding and awareness of similarities and differences between the therapist and the client.

In the last phase of the model, either by way of simulated lab experiences or actual direct client contact hours, trainees are tasked to reflect on how their knowledge and access to self can be *used as a clinical resource*. For example, if a white cis-gendered woman is working with a black cis-gendered client whose chief complaint is sexism in the workplace, the therapist may have little to no issue in addressing the impact of sexism and misogyny due to lived experience; however, the therapist who received this training would readily be able to access where and when they may be avoiding the topic of race (e.g., a sensory reaction and discomfort that inspires one to avoid the subject). The POTT model would assist the therapist to lean into the discomfort of race and make it a focal point of treatment which would lessen the burden on the black cis-gendered client to bring it up in treatment.

Trainees are given a multitude of opportunities to practice these types of scenarios in this last leg of the training. Currently, we use a live actor in the third phase of the model, and ask students to use their signature themes as the primary theory of therapy. Said another way, the humanity of the therapist is artfully used to develop a strong therapeutic alliance. We believe in providing students with this learning opportunity, as other courses will give focus to more formal theories of change that have less to do with the self as resource. In other words, they will learn about theoretical interventions elsewhere. In POTT, they learn that their unique relationship, that includes their unique personhood (each student is necessarily different), is a central pathway for clinical wellness.

We believe that the task of ethical development should not be arrested at the memorization of laws and professional codes. Instead, trainees deserve robust opportunities to navigate ethical considerations in action and in practice. These include instances where we can practice centering the narratives of people of color in therapy, having direct conversation, and deconstructing white supremacy norms in therapeutic practice. As such, the POTT model can be viewed as a proactive clinical training tool; a paradigm that underscores all of the ways we show up with our clients and their systems. Trainees can navigate ethical challenges well when they are given opportunities to develop knowledge of self, access to their own experiences, and skills training that follows.

Overall, across both of our careers, we feel we have been taught not to invite who we are into what we do, nor entertain the fact that our lived experiences are tools that can assist in client wellness and change. In our experiences, the personhood of a therapist is often seen as a separate domain from core curriculum. For example, both of us have had to create opportunities for person of the therapist reflections in the graduate school we currently work in, where self-work felt previously disjointed. We heard this from students, but also felt it ourselves; we will speak later to why this was the case, in our estimation, and what POTT can do to bring things together.

3   Who We Are

Confidence…It's you, a man on top of the hills.
  An individual, when hurt is all he feels,
  but on this confidence appeals,
  to the brain and the soul like emotional meals…

- • an excerpt from poem written by Zain Shamoon in 2005

3.1   Who Is Professor Zain Shamoon?

For me (Zain Shamoon, PhD), growing up in Southeast Michigan, the tokenism of non-white bodies was a driving force in my developmental experiences, especially in late childhood and early adolescent years. For many of those years, I had not considered my cultural identity as a Muslim American and South Asian person in a proactive way. Rather, my experiences of my own cultural being were more reactive within a largely white city, where I began to experience discrimination from peers in first grade. This trend followed through high school as well. I would be cast into a position to react to the white mass who made comments about brown people smelling bad, or off-key jokes that blended terrorism with Islam. In response, I would take pride in my cultural being, to respond to the haters, so to speak. However, it was not always safe to explore myself fully in a way that was not simply responsive to others' prejudices. I needed support and a sense of community to help me actualize cultural pride. While I had some of this, I continued to cope mostly in isolation. I mention all of this to say that one of the most powerful experiences for my sense of self was when I learned how to proactively engage in my cultural self, including curiosities that were for my own investment of self-knowledge, rather than to hold ground only when someone was emotionally attacking me about my identity.

Thus came a time of personal renaissance, starting in high school, when I started writing poetry in my bedroom. Looking back on these writings now, I see so much there about personal advocacy, community advocacy, and embracing my faith system of Islam with deep pride. At the time, I am sure a lot of my focus was on the formal qualities of poems, prose, and the use of effective rhyme schemes. However, as I scan the words from these poems now, I see how much wisdom was extracted from proactive self-exploration. I chose to sit down and write those pieces for myself. It was an act of self-love and cultural resistance against dominant forces of oppression.

Flashing forward several years, this was very similar to my experience of entering the field of family therapy. I had for many years chased achievement to please my parents, but to also quiet the white gaze upon which I was expected to be a model minority: an excellent student to ensure my place in the white man's hierarchy. However, I later discovered human ecological theory (Bronfenbrenner, 1986) in an entry level family therapy course. Here, something very freeing was unlocked in me: I began to develop an investment in how multiple layers of society acted upon each other to create pathways of development, or conversely constraints to human development. It felt like breathing; I had an academic language that fit so beautifully with how I saw the maze of life. In other words, my professional world became immersed with my personal development, a blend that I now see immersed within the person of the therapist (POTT) model (Aponte & Kissil, 2014) we will speak more about in this chapter. My hope for the field of family therapy is that we protect systems thinking, so that the multiple forces that act upon our development can be acknowledged. People deserve to be seen, heard, and supported, and systems thinkers with cultural humility are uniquely positioned to keep pushing the field forward this way. In our view, trainees deserve to experience humanity in the work we do as therapists.

3.2   Who Is Professor Anthony Pennant?

I (Anthony Pennant, PhD) am the first to achieve many things in my family, and that is one of the many identities that shape me. I am a first-generation American who is strongly rooted in the rich ethnic, racial, and social blending of the Caribbean. My father and his family are from Jamaica where the air is sweet, the way of life is to relax, and connection to family is everything. My father's family is, much like Jamaica, a melting pot of races, ethnicities, and customs that come from all walks of life, namely, Asian (Dravidian and Vietnamese peoples), African (Nigerian and Sierra Leonean), White/Caucus (Welsh and British), and Indigenous (Taino peoples) ancestry. I embrace each and every racial/ethnic part of my genealogy; however, I exist in a paradigm of society that wishes to reduce the wealth and diversity of my background to a physical representation that is solely based on my skin and color. I am forced to choose between how to identify as a Black person and reduce who I am.

To add to the complexity of who I am, another identity that plays a role in how I show up is my sexuality. I am a queer person but most readily share that I am a same-gender loving individual. Navigating sexual preference in and of itself has dangers which require me to constantly measure who, where, when, and what is safe for me to engage. This same dynamic exists for me being a person of color. When you add the totality of who I am, there is no escaping that I am not a White, heterosexual, cis-gendered male, and that I feel this in all environments. The combinations of who I am are hard to hold and often in competition. Being a person of color in the LGBT+ community does not prevent me from experiencing racism, which is why people of color like myself often protect ourselves from racial discrimination and/or microaggressions from members of the very same community.

4 Our Professional Convictions

Having introduced ourselves as individuals, we would like to continue our discussion with you regarding how we propose to shift the intention of family therapy in the following ways:

1. Transform training experiences so that they are truly centered on the lived experiences of diverse populations.
2. Decenter Eurocentric ideals of wellness in theoretical understandings and interventions.
3. Embrace the entirety of a therapist's personhood, as it is present in the therapeutic encounter with clients, as opposed to the therapist being a "blank slate."

We engage in this conversation as people of Color (POC) who are university professors who both hold advanced degrees. We are focused on altering the landscape in our field, to make room for the experiences of POC students/trainees in a central way, rather than as an afterthought or niche subject. We call for the field of Marriage and Family Therapy to transform how we think about and train clinicians to treat diverse individuals, relational units of various constellations, and families.

Prior to delving into the formal aspects of implementing POTT, it is important to discuss why we think this matters so much. As such, we will detail here the following matters: a) calling for *true systems* thinking that includes third-order change (McDowell et al., 2019); b) advocating for a sense of professional community; c) calling for family therapists to engage in community work, d) advocating for clinical learning/training to be embodied rather than a series of conceptual understandings; e) the importance of resisting status quo scripts about what makes a successful clinician; and f) reclaiming the humanity of our field, that once included a greater call for "here and now" moments in training and in therapy sessions (Minuchin et al., 2021).

5 When POTT Hits Home

In the following section of this chapter, we detail what stands out to us the most about the POTT model, and how this includes the embrace of therapist humanity, and an enhancement of sociocultural attunement for therapists. To date, our experiences of implementing POTT as teachers and therapists has meant: a transformation in how we conduct family therapy specifically, a deep consideration of colleague-ship in our careers, enhanced pathways to third-order change, and the development of sensory self-awareness.

5.1   Family Therapy and Sociocultural Attunement

To date, I (ZS) have been working with clients for over 13 years. One of the most difficult things for me to process, looking back at my first decade, is that I have not met that many clinicians who apply systems thinking beyond the family unit. That is, I meet many professionals who care about intergenerational family therapy, genograms, triangulations, and a host of dynamics that apply to family life. However, when called to task in directly attending to third-order matters, such as institutional racism, financial barriers to entry in therapy, larger curriculum changes across graduate schools (that also center the experiences of people from the global majority), I have only met a few people who hold this conviction in effect.

I want to stress this phrase "in effect"; there are many people who can speak to the third-order sociocultural matters I just spoke to, but whether or not their professional lives center these matters in action/in effect is another subject. For example, I have worked in two institutions (one as a graduate-student instructor, and one as a full-time professor) where diversity and inclusion statements were part of the mission statement, not only for the universities at large, but also within the departments within which I worked. However, when it came to conversations about centering immigrant student experiences while they were taking a diversity course, for example, I often felt alone in my convictions.

These gaps have often left me pining for a sense of collaborative company with others who care about third-order change. I have found, on rare occasions, the professional company of other faculty of color who hold these convictions, not only in their sentiments but also in their clinical work. My co-author, Dr. Anthony Pennant, is one such person, though my first encounter with folks who center third-order change was within the American Association for Marriage and Family Therapy Minority Fellowship program (MFP). It was there that I heard about the work that students were doing at Drexel University, where Harry Aponte's Person of the Therapist (Aponte & Kissil, 2014) model was uniquely flourishing. I came to understand that there was a way to do this work, in improving the mental health well-being of families in diverse communities, that was not centered on the latest popular therapy model at the status quo graduate school. My colleagues in the MFP were doing clinical work in prisons, or creating research about marginalized populations, or considering the lived experiences and needs of immigrant communities. As will be discussed in the next section, this experience taught me my first lesson in keeping good company in the field of family therapy, especially if under normal circumstances one is left feeling isolated without this.

5.2 Keeping Good Company

One of my (ZS) favorite components of the POTT model (Aponte & Kissil, 2014) is the opportunity it gives students/trainees to be with each other for a considerable period of time. At Antioch University Seattle, we utilize a cohort model so that students can be witnesses to each others' personal and professional growth process for at least 9 months (three quarters of coursework). The reason that this provides me satisfaction is that the opportunity to be *with* professional others has felt rare to me in my career (ZS). I remember being a graduate student and being told by professors that the markers of successful family therapists are two-fold: to be a tenured professor in a Commission on Accreditation for Marriage and Family Therapy accredited program and/or to create a lucrative private practice. In my estimation, either of these tracks can be quite isolating unless one is intentional about creating a network of support. I had felt this isolation already as a graduate student at Michigan State University, even though I am quite social and extroverted. That is because each of us was required to carry our own burdens with regard to research, publication, clinical work, and classroom competency. I remember feeling constantly flooded in stress, with a lack of sleep, and enduring times spent alone without others with whom I could touch base. I hope that in writing this, those with similar experiences can feel validated.

I recall times of contrasting relief marked by comradery and the opportunity to commiserate about these challenges with another colleague. POTT ensures this comradery (Lutz & Irizarry, 2009). My experience (ZS) is that for therapists of color who aspire to become tenured professors, the "table" is already filled with white men, and, without adequate support, one's cultural self can disappear. I have experienced this myself, often working as part of mostly white teams in academia, research, or clinics. We must recruit people in our programs from across cultures, with different perspectives and sensibilities, in order to enrich the field.

Enriching the community through keeping good company is a challenge to the status quo of isolated realities. This sense of connection was a lifeline for me when I was able to experience connection with professional others in the MFP, and recently at Antioch University Seattle with a shift to more professors of color in our department. Of course, I have also felt this connection with Anthony in our shared work with the POTT model in training and teaching together. However, I do not feel that this is commonplace.

We (ZS and AP) hope to underscore this benefit of comradery in our application of the POTT model; that we grow professionally and personally in the company of others (by contrast to the hyper-individualistic goals one "should" be meeting). I view this as a battle between the cultural self who knows that community matters, versus the problem-saturated narrative (White & Epston, 1990) that creates a thin story about what success looks like. I hope to use my career, including by way of the POTT model, to advocate for clinicians keeping good professional company.

5.3   The Call for Community Work: Third-Order Change

Another way professionals in the field of family therapy can keep from experiencing isolation is for therapists to be engaged in their communities. The major benefit in doing this beyond curtailing isolation, however, is the ability to spread mental health healing beyond our therapy rooms. In our view, if we are to truly embrace systems thinking, especially systemic perspectives that include attention to the wellness of various communities who cannot readily access therapy, then working out in the community is an imperative.

Given this, in the second quarter of student training, Dr. Pennant and I have stressed the importance of third order change (McDowell et al., 2019). Week to week, we engage our students in dialogue about how to achieve that third-order change. In having these discussions over the past 2 years across three POTT cohorts, students have provided many examples of how this may be achieved. For example, some have shared the importance of universities giving back financially to indigenous populations beyond simply giving a land acknowledgment. Others have discussed the importance of advocating for affordable therapy services, sliding scales, and therapy appointments that occur past 5 pm to accommodate families who cannot come during the daytime. Others have discussed the importance of Licensed Marriage and Family Therapist (LMFT) reciprocity across states, especially in a time when telehealth is becoming more regular, so that moving states does not have to mean losing your therapist.

These pathways and discussions can only be promoted when we are talking about third-order change more regularly in our classrooms and in other family therapy training settings. Our second quarter of POTT training for students at Antioch University Seattle was designed to promote exactly this, and this type of learning is not something we have personally witnessed often. Students in our POTT training are invited to discuss how community work, volunteership, and third-order change are part of their signature themes: their patterned ways of relating to the world that they can embrace and use for good. In the first quarter, POTT signature themes are discussed with reference to family-of-origin dynamics primarily. The second quarter moves to more active discussion about sociocultural attunement, which is an integral part of our definition of true systems thinking (ZS and AP).

6 Touchpoints of Self: Sensory Self-Knowledge

In Aponte's POTT model, one of three crucial training components is called *Access to Self* (Aponte & Kissil, 2014). We have already discussed how community engagement can be a way to practice the story of one's signature theme (and one's clinical identity). During the second quarter of the POTT-training, we invite students to practice other ways of accessing themselves. Said another way, students deserve to *feel, embody,* and *experience* their training, especially as client cases will inspire a wide range of emotional responses and sensory experiences for the therapist. Static data points in a medical chart are not the same as the *happening* of therapy. As such, we believe that students/trainees deserve to have practice sitting with their "access" touchpoints. For example, one can ask, "Where does one feel it on their body when they feel anxious?" Or they might ask, "Where do you sense it on your person when you don't understand a client or feel incompetent in the moment? How does it feel when you feel rewarded by a session with a client? How does your body let you know when you had a good moment in therapy with your clients?"

We practice these types of "access" curiosities during POTT training in an ongoing way. This defies the western sensibility to first rationalize, think, and then act. Instead, it centers the body and sensory knowledge of people as a core site of knowledge and action. Years ago, I (ZS) had a case with a client who had been making cuts on her arms to harm herself. She was highly depressed, felt socially isolated, and was having constant family conflict. I felt a strong sense of care for this client, in part because she had similar sociocultural identities as I do. My client was South Asian, Muslim, and had been struggling with self-defeatism, as I had in my teen and young adult years. As part of an effort to be "competent," I linked concepts from her case file to her family history in an effort to inform her about her own situation. But, she did not need my help with this! She was already living her life, and she did not need me explaining *who she was* to her.

I went to my supervisor, Kathleen Burns-Jager (one of the greatest clinicians I have ever known and had the pleasure to work with) to ask her advice about the impasse I was feeling in this case. I explained that this client would come in for a string of sessions, disappear for a while, call in suddenly under duress to make another appointment, and then repeat this cycle over and over. It was clear she was playing out some relational themes with me that she had likely experienced elsewhere.

In response to the predicament I shared, Kathleen asked me something I will always remember. Paraphrasing her words, she asked me to consider what it would be like to tell my client how *I was feeling* in the session. Immediately all of my socialized red flags from western academia went off in flares. I thought, "that's me centering myself, she's going to leave the sessions and never come back. Yet something in me resonated with Kathleen's wisdom, so I gave it a try. My next session, I told the client that I noticed she had periods when she came in, and then I didn't see her for a while, and then she came back in a panic. I told her I was concerned about this pattern. Even though a part of me questioned my decision to disclose this, I also felt a sense of authenticity in sharing this with her. I actually think I felt it in my stomach (this is where I have always felt my most intense emotions; this is where I can *access* my signature theme). After trusting that place and making this move, I was delighted when the client replied "yeah, I know I do that." It was a de-mystifying moment in therapy for both of us, and it humanized the sessions going forward. In effect, humanizing the session created a new homeostasis for me and the client to work with.

I learned then and there that prioritizing shared humanity, slowing down, and artfully self-disclosing (using the sensory experience as a catalyst) can be more useful than concepts and theories depending on the case. This of course relates to the importance of the therapeutic alliance (Blow et al., 2007) in achieving positive outcomes, no matter what theoretical model is being used.

Students/trainees deserve to practice access to self, acknowledging what is happening for them in the moment of the therapeutic encounter with clients. This is where they can learn to *feel it all*, as well as learn how to use those feelings therapeutically! After all, therapy, in our estimation, is not just a social "science." It is also an actionable art form; a sensibility about mental health known more readily in other cultures who do not necessarily prioritize "mind over matter," but rather center what it means to *sit with* someone in their struggles. We strongly believe that this is at the core of the POTT model: to sit with someone in their humanity. We are excited to center this type of learning for trainees, students, and colleagues, for the rest of our careers.

7   Resisting the Status Quo Script

Unfortunately, over the past several years, we have experienced our fair share of field resistance to these proposed shifts in training. For example, we recently experienced the resistance of a colleague who patronized our shift to center the experiences of non-white students in POTT quarter two (this is also the multicultural perspectives course at Antioch University Seattle). She often questioned us about why more people of color needed to be hired, or whether or not the work we were doing was thoughtful enough of "other" intersections. We have rarely seen this concern lofted upon white professors. Needless to say, this was a white member of academia who seemed to be having a hard time witnessing people of color add something to the field. We had witnessed this colleague engage in the same type of top-down discussions with other faculty of color.

The killing of George Floyd in 2020, as well as social resistance to a series of murders on black bodies, made matters worse for many of us in academia. We observed white faculty members from multiple disciplines who retreated from discussions about cultural sensitivity in academia, and even avoided engaging with students of color on campus. Our work has been impeded by encountering these people who have attempted to derail or distract from conversations about race. Back to isolation for us, right? Are we being asked by our white colleagues to revert back to working in our own little pocket, as isolated professionals? Thankfully, folks like Dr. Jennifer Sampson, Dr. Alba Niño, Dr. Cayla Minaiy, Dr. Adrian Blow, and Jay Lappin have encouraged us to keep going. Now, we proudly defy the status quo about what is "good science"; new pathways are needed.

8   Reclaiming the Field

When I (ZS) was a master's student at Michigan State, the final thesis in the couple and family therapy (CFT) department involved an oral presentation about our theory of change. I remember feeling a strong alignment with experiential therapy and narrative therapy at that time. I have since reflected upon this choice I made back then, and can see a stark difference between myself and the "evidenced-based" culture of the time. It was an expectation of our professors that we understood the state of the field, the importance of the Gottmans, the importance of Susan Johnson, and the dominance of cognitive behavioral therapy (CBT). In other words, I got the loud and clear message to follow what was famous, and to align with what other professors across different universities would see as acceptable. I have no misgivings about the importance of the people I mentioned and their contributions. At the same time it is not lost on me that I was being socialized to see my professional North Star in alignment with white theorists. Fortunately or unfortunately, I am a rabble rouser; my father taught me to resist when I observed mixed-up priorities in any institution. That is exactly how I felt then, and that is how I feel now – the priorities are mixed up in our field. I feel now, as I did then, that the humanity of therapy sessions should always matter more than what is popular, because what is popular will change. Being able to *sit with* clients is an ever-present conviction we should all have as therapists. When I go to a therapist, I want my therapist to tend to my life, instead of being anxious about their own competence next to what is "in."

I think what allowed me to do my master's presentation differently from this expectation was that I was in awe of the work I saw from Virginia Satir (Rasheed et al., 2010). The tradition of "here and now" moments of therapy extends beyond her in a deep stratosphere that includes people like Harry Aponte, Carmen Knudson-Martin (Knudson-Martin et al., 2021), and Salvador Minuchin (Minuchin et al., 2021).

A few years later, I re-read the Autobiography of Malcolm X (Malcolm & Haley, 1966). Besides reading this again for personal reasons, I was struck by the community-based program he had created for those suffering from substance abuse/dependency. This highly productive program of rehabilitation from substance use included community check-ins, former addicts spending time with current addicts, and round the clock support from one's social support system. Perhaps this type of work was not mainstream because it was *too black; too Muslim* (since the American psyche was scared of black Muslims). Unless embraced by the status quo or later culturally appropriated in an "adaptation" study by a well-known white professor, in my opinion, such legacies are viewed as niche and "out there." Could this also be a reason for Harry Aponte's lack of academic recognition? Is it not white enough for academia to embrace it?

9   Here and Now Theorists

In our view, it should not be assumed that therapists simply know how to attune to "the contextual here and now," and that they effectively know to use these moments wisely in the service of client healing. For example, much has been debated about whether or not therapists should use self-disclosure as a resource in therapy (Roberts, 2005). However, we argue that therapists using any aspect of self, including artful disclosure, should do so by first attuning toward themselves. Therapist anxiety and projections are an inevitability (Shamoon et al., 2017) because we too are human beings with unresolved tensions carried inside. We might be reminded of this in any moment of the therapeutic encounter. As such, taking what we know about the value of experiences (Rasheed et al., 2010) and attending to the here and now (Minuchin et al., 2021), it is important to carry forward the legacy of Harry Aponte and colleagues, who called on the field to embrace personal development for the "wounded healer," so that we have more attuned and mindful therapists in the field.

10 Conclusion: Moving from Systemic Thinking to Systemic Training (Isomorphism)

The field of family therapy, as a fundamentally systemic science and practice, is well suited to continue supporting the development and healing of the global majority, including historically oppressed communities. The POTT model provides assurance that trainees will self-reflect on how their own personhood impacts therapy. In doing so, trainees engage with their responsibility to create an environment of active and ongoing cultural sensitivity in the therapy room.

As we hope you have observed in reading our personal stories, POTT is an opportunity to call further attention to narratives of the oppressed, their identities, and pathways to healing. We are interested in furthering this type of clinical training that centers these stories in an embodied way. We invite the field of family therapy to embrace sociocultural systems thinking as the core feature of the field. The POTT model is the way we can practice this reclamation.

References

Aponte, H. J., & Kissil, K. (2014). "If I can grapple with this I can truly be of use in the therapy room": Using the therapist's own emotional struggles to facilitate effective therapy. *Journal of Marital and Family Therapy, 40*(2), 152–164. https://doi.org/10.1111/jmft.12011

Blow, A. J., Sprenkle, D. H., & Davis, S. D. (2007). Is who delivers the treatment more important than the treatment itself? The role of the therapist in common factors. *Journal of Marital and Family Therapy, 33*(3), 298–317. https://doi.org/10.1111/j.1752-0606.2007.00029.x

Bronfenbrenner, U. (1986). Ecology of the family as a context for human development: Research perspectives. *Developmental Psychology, 22*(6), 723–742. https://doi.org/10.1037/0012-1649.22.6.723

Knudson-Martin, C., Kim, L., Gibbs, E., & Harmon, R. (2021). Sociocultural attunement to vulnerability in couple therapy: Fulcrum for changing power processes. *Family Process, 60*, 1152–1169. https://doi.org/10.1111/famp.12635

Lutz, L., & Irizarry, S. S. (2009). Reflections of two trainees: Person-of-the-therapist training for couple and family therapists. *Journal of Marital and Family Therapy, 35*(4), 370–380. https://doi.org/10.1111/j.1752-0606.2009.00126.x

Malcolm, X., & Haley, A. (1966). *The autobiography of Malcolm X*. Grove Press.

McDowell, T., Knudson-Martin, C., & Bermudez, M. (2019). Toward third thinking in family therapy: Addressing social justice across family therapy practice. *Family Process, 58*, 9–22. https://doi.org/10.1111/famp.12383

Minuchin, S., Reiter, M. D., & Borda, C. (2021). *The craft of family therapy: Challenging certainties*. Routledge.

Rasheed, J. M., Rasheed, M. N., Rasheed, M. N., & Marley, J. A. (2010). *Family therapy: Models and techniques*. SAGE.

Roberts, J. (2005). Transparency and self-disclosure in family therapy: Dangers and possibilities. *Family Process, 44*(1), 45–63. https://doi.org/10.1111/j.1545-5300.2005.00041.x

Shamoon, Z. A., Lappan, S., & Blow, A. J. (2017). Managing anxiety: A therapist common factor. *Contemporary Family Therapy, 39*(1), 43–53. https://doi.org/10.1007/s10591-016-9399-1

White, M., & Epston, D. (1990). Narrative means to therapeutic ends. W.W. Norton & Company.

Index

A
Accountability, 2, 5, 14–16, 19, 41, 45–46, 59, 60, 72
Anti-racism, 7, 64, 66–70, 72, 73
Antiracist, 85–95

B
Bibliotherapy, 81, 82

C
Clinical education, 79–82
Co-teaching, 13–25
Couple and family therapy, 23, 63–74, 86, 108
Cultural attunement, 77–83
Cultural diversity, 13, 92
Culture, 3, 4, 6, 7, 17, 30, 32, 34, 39, 46, 60–62, 72, 80, 87, 94, 97, 104, 107, 108
Curriculum, 4, 7, 23, 35, 62, 69–72, 88, 91, 99, 103

D
Doctoral program, 17, 63, 86

E
Education, 10, 27–38, 41, 45, 50, 63, 64, 66, 78, 79, 85–95

F
Faculty of color, 2, 13, 14, 22, 23, 66, 69, 70, 73, 103, 108
Family therapy, 2, 24, 27, 31, 33, 40, 70, 77, 78, 87, 97, 100–105, 110
Family therapy education, 30

M
Macro-aggressions, 39, 73, 86
Marriage and family therapy, 7, 8, 31, 49, 50, 77, 78, 83, 86
Mentorship, 52–53, 57, 85–95
Microaggressions, 29, 56, 57, 61, 64, 73, 90, 92, 93, 102

P
Pedagogy, 23, 33, 85–95